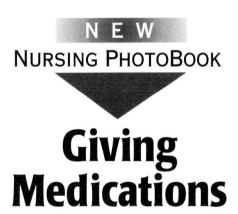

NEW
NURSING PHOTOBOOK

Giving Medications

NEW

NURSING PHOTOBOOK

Giving Medications

Springhouse Corporation
Springhouse, Pennsylvania

STAFF

Senior Publisher
Matthew Cahill

Clinical Manager
Cindy Tryniszewski, RN, MSN

Art Director
John Hubbard

Senior Editor
June Norris

Clinical Editors
Judith Schilling McCann, RN, BSN (clinical project editor), Beverly Tscheschlog, RN

Editor
Elizabeth Weinstein

Copy Editors
Cynthia C. Breuninger (manager), Lynette High, Doris Weinstock

Designers
Stephanie Peters (senior associate art director), Lorraine Carbo, Darcy Feralio

Photographer
John Gallagher

Typographers
Diane Paluba (manager), Elizabeth Bergman, Joyce Rossi Biletz, Phyllis Marron, Valerie Rosenberger

Manufacturing
Deborah Meiris (director), Pat Dorshaw (manager), T.A. Landis

Production Coordinator
Margaret A. Rastiello

Editorial Assistants
Beverly Lane, Mary Madden

Indexer
Barbara Hodgson

©1996 by Springhouse Corporation. All rights reserved. No part of this publication may be used or reproduced in any manner whatsoever without written permission except for brief quotations embodied in critical articles and reviews. For information, write Springhouse Corporation, 1111 Bethlehem Pike, P.O. Box 908, Springhouse, PA 19477-0908. Authorization to photocopy items for internal or personal use, or for the internal or personal use of specific clients, is granted by Springhouse Corporation for users registered with the Copyright Clearance Center (CCC) Transactional Reporting Service, provided that the fee of $.75 per page is paid directly to CCC, 27 Congress St., Salem, MA 01970. For those organizations that have been granted a license by CCC, a separate system of payment has been arranged. The fee code for users of the Transactional Reporting Service is 0874348129/96 $00.00 + $.75. Printed in the United States of America

A member of the Reed Elsevier plc group

PHOBK5-010795

Library of Congress Cataloging-in-Publication Data
Giving medications.
    p. cm. — (New nursing photobooks)
Includes index.
    1. Drugs—Administration.   2. Nursing.
I. Springhouse Corporation.   II. Series
[DNLM: 1. Drugs—administration & dosage.
WB 340 G539 1996]
RM147.G576   1996
615'.6—dc20
DNLM/DLC   95-11492
ISBN 0-87434-812-9   CIP

CONTENTS

FOREWORD

The rapid development of new drugs and the introduction of increasingly complex delivery systems have dramatically increased the role of drug therapy in health care. One of our most demanding jobs as nurses is administering medications safely and monitoring their effectiveness.

With this responsibility in mind, you'll want to keep a copy of *Giving Medications* close at hand. This book is designed to help you administer today's medications accurately and safely. You'll appreciate the step-by-step photographs that walk you through 25 methods of giving drugs. Using large, detailed photographs accompanied by simple, concisely written instructions, *Giving Medications* explains every important technique for giving medications.

Two characteristics make this book invaluable: its comprehensive coverage and its applicability and accessibility to every user. Recognizing that your responsibilities change virtually from day to day, the clinical experts who created this book provide directions for giving drugs through a wide range of routes, including oral and topical, transdermal, S.C., and I.M. You'll find photographs on giving drugs through tubes and through a secondary I.V. line, assisting with intrapleural injections, and more. You can stay current on new methods, such as implanting a drug into the abdomen, giving a needle-free injection, giving insulin through an implanted catheter, and using a retractable needle and syringe.

Whether you need a fast review of instilling nasal drugs or a complete lesson on delivering drugs with a syringe pump, *Giving Medications* is equally easy to use. The book is divided into two major sections: "Administering Oral and Topical Drugs" and "Giving Injections and Infusions." You can quickly find what you need.

To help increase your proficiency, look for the special graphic devices, or logos, that signal key features. *Clinical tips* provide quick insight into special situations or tell you how to perform steps more efficiently. *Troubleshooting* charts outline equipment problems and how to keep them from happening again. In *Complications* charts, you'll find indispensable information on potential patient hazards; for example, when delivering insulin with an infusion pump.

As nursing moves into the 21st century, don't let the promise of increasingly high-tech drug delivery systems intimidate you. Just make sure you pick the right resources to inform and guide you. I can't recommend a more valuable resource than *Giving Medications*.

Mary Jo Gerlach, RN, MSNEd
Assistant Professor, Adult Nursing
Medical College of Georgia
School of Nursing, Athens

Administering Oral and Topical Drugs

LEARNING ABOUT DRUG ADMINISTRATION

Administration of drugs may seem like a routine nursing task. However, it carries the twin responsibilities of ensuring the patient's safety and maximizing the drug's therapeutic effect. To meet these responsibilities, you need to know the indications, normal dosage, therapeutic and adverse effects, and potential interactions of every drug you administer. You'll also need to be familiar with pharmacokinetics: how a drug is absorbed, distributed, metabolized, and excreted. (See *Quick guide to pharmacokinetics,* page 4.)

GIVING DRUGS CORRECTLY

You'll need to assess your patient each time you administer a drug. You'll do this to ensure that the patient's condition hasn't changed to an extent that would contraindicate continuing drug therapy. To further protect the patient, observe the five "rights" of drug administration, as described below.

Right name

Check to make sure that the name, room number, and bed number on the medication record match the information on the patient's identification bracelet. And don't just ask the patient to verify his name. If he doesn't hear you correctly or if he's confused, he may agree to a name that's not his.

Right drug

Make sure that the drug you're about to administer is the same drug the doctor ordered. Because some drugs have similar names, be alert for transcription errors. Is the action of the drug you're administering applicable to the patient's condition? If not, notify the patient's doctor.

  Check the label on the medication package three times: when you take it from the shelf or the patient's medication drawer, when you dispense the drug or open the unit-dose pack, and again as you return the medication container to its proper place or as you discard the unit-dose wrapper.

Right dose

Double-check that the dose you're giving is the same dose that the doctor ordered. Is it within the usual range? If not, verify the dose by checking the original order or by asking the doctor.

Right route

Make sure that the route you're about to use is the same route ordered by the doctor. Ask yourself, "Is this the usual route for this drug? Does this particular drug, or the selected route, require any special administration techniques?" For instance, to prevent tissue staining, I.M. iron must be given using the Z-track technique and oral iron should be given through a straw.

Right time and frequency

Verify that you're administering the drug at the appropriate time and frequency. Consider the actions of the drug and how they may affect the time of administration. For example, administering a diuretic at night will interfere with the patient's sleep.

Other considerations

Besides these "rights" that help ensure safe administration, you must consider the patient's rights. The patient, for instance, has a right to know why he's getting a drug and which adverse effects to expect. And he has the right to refuse medication.

  Never give a drug that someone else has prepared, and remember to dispose of any unused medication properly. Also, if the patient questions you about a particular drug or dosage, stop administering the drug immediately. Then recheck the medication record, the doctor's order, and the patient's identification bracelet to ensure that everything is correct before you continue.

ORAL DRUG FORMS

Oral administration is the most convenient and economical way of delivering medication to the body. It's also the most commonly used route for many drugs. Oral drug forms include tablets, enteric-coated tablets, capsules, syrups, elixirs, oils, liquids, suspensions, powders, and granules. The absorption rate for each drug form depends on how the drug dissolves before passing to the small intestine. For example, special coatings on some drugs delay dissolution and, thereby, absorption. (See *How the GI tract absorbs drugs,* page 5.)

  As you give oral medications to your patient, keep in mind ways to overcome a drug's unpleasant taste. (See *Enhancing palatability,* page 5.)

Joanne Patzek DaCunha, RN, MSN, who contributed to this section, is the associate clinical director at Springhouse Corporation. The publisher also thanks the following organizations for their help: *Doylestown (Pa.) Hospital; Grand View Hospital,* Sellersville, Pa.; *Hill Rom,* Batesville, Ind.; *Sherwood Medical,* St Louis, Mo.; *Village Pharmacy,* Springhouse, Pa.

Quick guide to pharmacokinetics

When a drug enters the body, it must be absorbed into the central circulation and distributed to its site of action. For its action to stop, a drug must be metabolized and excreted along with any metabolites. Here's how this process works.

Absorption

Different routes or sites of administration affect drug absorption.

• *Mucous membranes.* Because mucous membranes are the thinnest, most vascular dermal surface, they usually transfer a drug into the bloodstream rapidly and effectively, although the extent of systemic absorption varies according to the administration site. Essentially, the mucous membranes absorb a drug by diffusion, infiltration, and osmosis.

• *GI tract.* Also called enteral administration, GI administration is safe, easy, and economical—even though GI absorption may sometimes be unpredictable. To be absorbed from the GI tract, a drug must be dissolved or in liquid form. Dissolution of a solid drug usually occurs in the stomach, with the extent of dissolution depending on the drug formulation, the pH of gastric fluids, the gastric contents, and the coating on the drug (some coatings prevent or slow breakdown in the stomach). Once dissolved, the drug passes to the small intestine, which has a large surface area, good blood supply, and a moderate pH, making it ideal for drug absorption.

• *Parenteral sites.* Whether the route is intradermal, subcutaneous, intramuscular, intra-arterial, intravenous, epidural, spinal, or intraosseous, parenteral administration facilitates rapid and reliable drug absorption. However, the extent of absorption varies among the routes. For example, the intradermal route is associated with the slowest absorption. The intramuscular route, by contrast, allows more rapid absorption because of the extensive blood supply in muscles and fasciae. By delivering the drug directly to the bloodstream, the intravenous and intra-arterial routes provide the fastest and most efficient absorption.

• *Respiratory tract.* By this route, small drug particles inhaled into the respiratory tract move to the alveoli, where they quickly cross the alveolocapillary membrane into the bloodstream. The respiratory tract's large surface area and generous blood supply enhance absorption. However, the extent of absorption varies with the rate and depth of respiration, the drug's particle size, and the drug's ability to move across the alveolocapillary membrane.

• *Skin.* Although most drugs applied to the skin are used only for local effect, absorption may occur if the skin is irritated or broken. Even with drugs designed to be delivered through the skin, the extent of absorption varies according to the thickness of the skin and the type of drug delivery device.

Distribution

After absorption, the drug circulates to its site of action. Only a free-circulating drug can cross cell membranes and enter body tissues. During distribution, some of the drug may reach and be stored in plasma protein, fat, and muscle. The extent of distribution depends on such factors as the lipid solubility of the drug, blood supply to body tissues, and membrane permeability.

Metabolism

To terminate drug action, various biological processes transform the drug into a more easily excreted form. Commonly called drug metabolism, this biotransformation occurs by two reactions: nonsynthetic and synthetic. Nonsynthetic reactions oxidize, hydrolyze, or reduce the drug. These reactions can occur in the liver or other tissues, such as the kidneys, lungs, plasma, or intestinal mucosa. Synthetic reactions occur in the liver, where hepatic enzymes conjugate, or join, the drug to other substances (such as glucuronic acid) to make the transformed drug molecules water-soluble and, thereby, more excretable. Of course, hepatic, renal, and cardiovascular disease can alter the rate and extent of biotransformation.

Excretion

A drug remains active until it's metabolized into an inactive substance or excreted. The kidneys handle most excretion by expelling both the drug and its metabolites. The excretion rate and efficiency depend on the adequacy of cardiovascular, hepatic, and renal function. Additional drug excretion may occur through the skin, lungs, feces, saliva, tears, and breast milk.

How the GI tract absorbs drugs

As shown in the photograph, the form of oral drugs determines where disintegration, dissolution, and absorption occur in the GI tract.

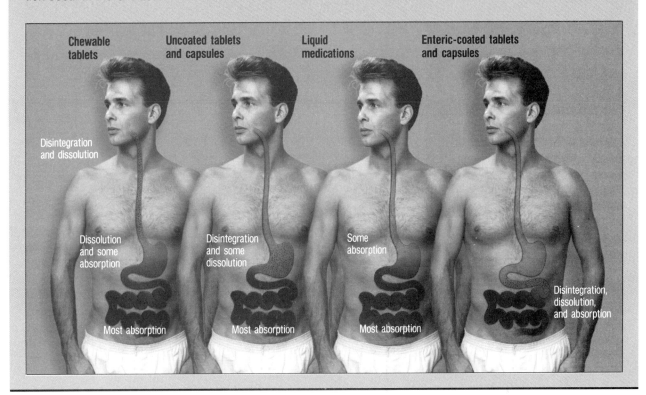

Chewable tablets
- Disintegration and dissolution
- Dissolution and some absorption
- Most absorption

Uncoated tablets and capsules
- Disintegration and some dissolution
- Most absorption

Liquid medications
- Some absorption
- Most absorption

Enteric-coated tablets and capsules
- Disintegration, dissolution, and absorption

Enhancing palatability

Some drugs, especially those in liquid or powder form, have an unpleasant taste. To promote patient compliance, consider these tips for disguising a drug's unpleasant taste.
- Mix the drug with fruit juice or cola syrup, if allowed. Have the patient sip the mixture through a straw.
- Use a syringe to instill the drug into the pocket between the patient's cheek and teeth.
- Suggest that the patient suck on ice chips just before taking the drug.
- Unless the patient is receiving a small amount of the drug, pour it over ice.
- Tell the patient to hold his nose as he swallows the drug.
- Chill oily medications.
- Offer a piece of hard candy or chewing gum after the patient swallows the drug, if allowed, or let him gargle or rinse his mouth.

GIVING ORAL DRUGS

To administer a drug orally, you'll need the patient's medication record; the ordered medication; a souffle cup or a plastic, graduated medicine cup; and gloves, if needed. Also obtain a glass of water or other liquid to help the patient swallow the medication. If you plan to crush a tablet, you'll need a mortar and pestle; to divide a scored tablet, you'll need a knife or scoring device and a paper towel. For measuring liquid medications, you'll also need a damp paper towel.

To administer liquid medication to an infant, collect the prescribed medication, a medicine dropper, and a bib.

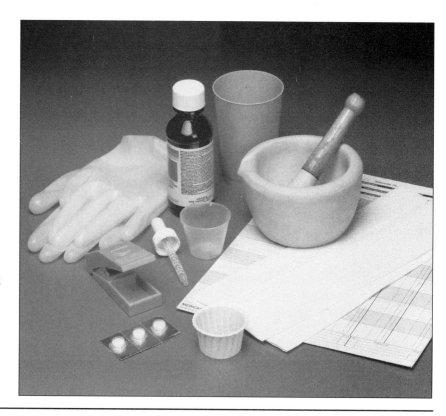

Giving tablets and capsules

First, wash your hands. Then remove the unit-dose tablet or capsule from the patient's medication drawer, or select the prescribed bottle of tablets or capsules from the shelf. Open the container and pour the required number of tablets or capsules into the container lid. If you pour too many, return the excess to the container without touching them. Next, place the correct number of tablets or capsules in the souffle cup (as shown).

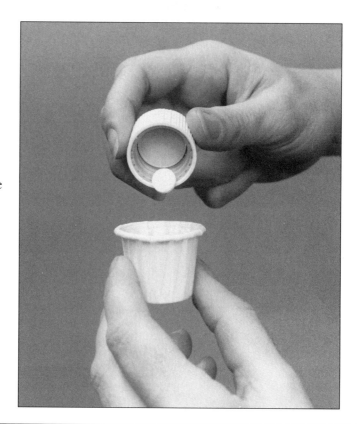

If you're using a unit-dose packet, open the wrapper and place the medication in the cup.

Note: If you're providing a chewable tablet, make sure that the patient chews it thoroughly before swallowing. Also, caution him not to chew other tablets, particularly coated ones.

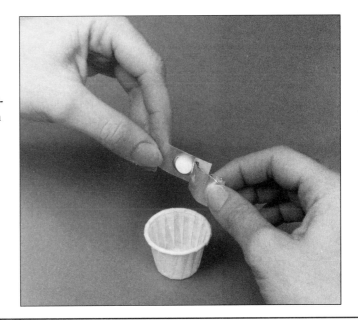

To crush a tablet, make sure that the mortar and pestle are clean and that no remnants from a previously crushed tablet remain. Then place the tablet in the mortar, and crush it completely with the pestle (as shown). Move the crushed tablet into a medicine cup or directly into the fluid or food in which it will be mixed. Remove all drug particles from the mortar.

▶ *Clinical tip:* To save time, use the pestle to crush the tablet in its unopened wrapper. Be sure to remove all the medication before discarding the wrapper.

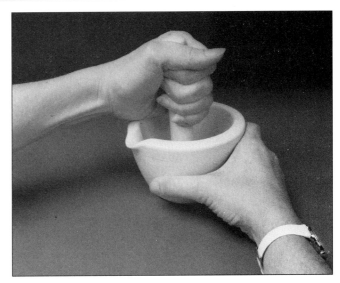

To split a scored tablet, use a paper towel to grab both sides of the tablet. Then push down on the edges to break it. If the tablet is difficult to break or if it isn't scored, use the knife or scoring device to make a small slit in the center of the tablet. To use the scoring device, place the tablet in the device (as shown) and close the lid. Then place the correct dose in the souffle cup, and properly discard the unused portion.

Next, check the patient's identification bracelet and administer the medication.

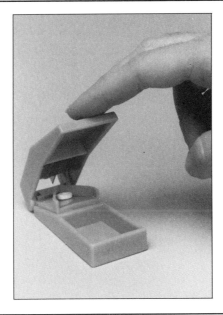 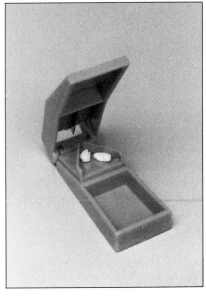

Dispensing liquid medication

Take the bottle from the patient's medication drawer or shelf. If the medication is in a suspension, shake it well. Then uncap the bottle, and place the cap upside down on a clean surface. Holding the graduated medicine cup at eye level, pour the correct amount of medication to the correct dose mark (as shown). Wipe the bottle lip with a damp paper towel and replace the cap.

Next, check the patient's identification bracelet and administer the medication with whichever liquid or food you've chosen to help him swallow.

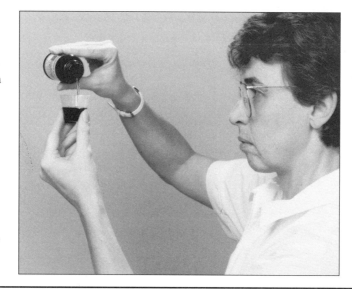

If you're giving an oral liquid medication to an infant, first put a bib under his chin. Then hold him securely. With your free hand, withdraw the correct amount of medication from the bottle by squeezing the bulb on the dropper. Hold the dropper at eye level to check the amount. Squeeze any excess medication into a sink or waste receptacle; don't return it to the bottle.

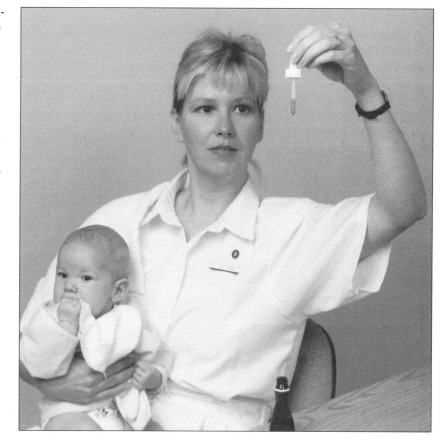

Hold the infant in the crook of your arm so that his head is elevated at a 45-degree angle. Gently instill the drops into his mouth. If the dropper isn't calibrated, hold it vertically over the infant's open mouth and instill the prescribed number of drops.

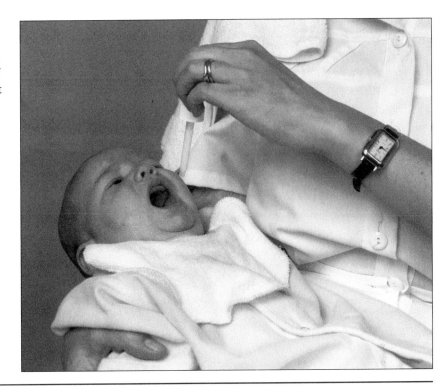

If you're using a calibrated dropper, instill the medication into the pocket between the infant's cheek and tongue (as shown here).

If the dropper touches the infant's mouth, wash the dropper thoroughly. Then return the dropper to the bottle and close it securely.

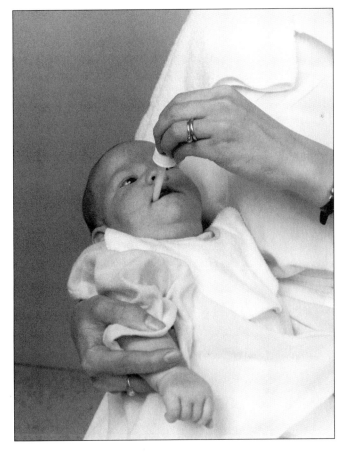

Drugs that mustn't be crushed or dissolved

When you're preparing solid drugs for administration, be careful not to crush or dissolve a drug if doing so can impair its effectiveness or absorption. Many drug forms (such as slow release, enteric coated, encapsulated beads, wax matrix, sublingual, buccal, and effervescent tablet preparations) are formulated to release their active ingredient for a specified duration or at a predetermined time after administration. Disrupting these formulations by crushing can dramatically affect the drug absorption rate and increase the risk of adverse effects.

Other reasons not to crush a drug involve such considerations as taste, tissue irritation, and unusual formulation—for example a capsule within a capsule, a liquid within a capsule, or a multiple, compressed tablet. Avoid crushing these drugs, which are listed here by brand name, for the reasons noted beside them.

Accutane (mucous membrane irritant)
Actifed 12-Hour (slow-release)
Acutrim (slow release)
Aerolate Sr., Jr., III (slow release)
Afrinol Repetabs (slow release)
Allerest 12 Hour (slow release)
Artane Sequels (slow release)
ASA Enseals (enteric coated)
Atrohist-LA
Atrohist Sprinkle (slow release)
Azulfidine EN-Tabs (enteric coated)
Bayer Timed-Release Arthritic Pain Formula (slow release)
Betapen-VK (taste)
Biphetamine (slow release)
Bisacodyl (enteric coated)
Bisco-Lax (enteric coated)
Bontril Slow-Release (slow release)
Breonesin (liquid filled)
Brexin L.A. (slow release)
Bromfed (slow release)
Bromfed-PD (slow release)
Calan SR (slow release)
Cama Arthritis Pain Reliever (multiple compressed tablet)
Carbiset-TR (slow release)
Cardizem (slow release)
Cardizem CD (slow release)
Cardizem-SR (slow release)
Carter's Little Pills (enteric coated)
Charcoal Plus (enteric coated)
Chloral Hydrate (liquid within a capsule)
Chlorpheniramine Maleate Time Release (slow release)
Chlor-Trimeton Repetabs (slow release)

Choledyl SA (slow release)
Cipro (taste)
Codimal-L.A. (slow release)
Colace (taste)
Comhist LA (slow release)
Compazine Spansule (slow release)
Congess SR, JR (slow release)
Constant-T (slow release)
Contac (slow release)
Cotazym-S (enteric coated)
Creon (enteric coated)
Dallergy (slow release)
Dallergy-D (slow release)
Dallergy-Jr. (slow release)
Deconamine SR (slow release)
Deconsal Sprinkle (slow release)
Deconsal II (slow release)
Demazin Repetabs (slow release)
Depakene (slow release, mucous membrane irritant)
Depakote (enteric coated)
Desoxyn Gradumet (slow release)
Desyrel (taste)
Dexedrine Spansule (slow release)
Diamox Sequels (slow release)
Dilatrate-SR (slow release)
Dimetane Extentabs (slow release)
Disobrom (slow release)
Disophrol Chronotabs (slow release)
Dital (slow release)
Donnatal Extentabs (slow release)
Donnazyme (enteric coated)
Drisdol (liquid filled)
Drixoral (slow release)
Drixoral Sinus (slow release)
Dulcolax (enteric coated)
Easprin (enteric coated)
Ecotrin (enteric coated)
E.E.S. 400 (enteric coated)

Elixophyllin SR (slow release)
E-Mycin (enteric coated)
Endafed (slow release)
Entex LA (slow release)
Entozyme (enteric coated)
Equanil (taste)
Ergostat (sublingual)
Eryc (enteric coated)
Ery-Tab (enteric coated)
Erythrocin Stearate (enteric coated)
Erythromycin Base (enteric coated)
Eskalith CR (slow release)
Fedahist Timecaps (slow release)
Feldene (mucous membrane irritant)
Feocyte (slow release)
Feosol (enteric coated)
Feosol Spansule (slow release)
Feratab (enteric coated)
Fergon (slow release)
Fero-Grad 500 mg (slow release)
Fero-Gradumet (slow release)
Ferralet SR (slow release)
Festal II (enteric coated)
Feverall Sprinkle Caps (taste)
Fumatinic (slow release)
Geocillin (taste)
Gris-PEG (crushing may cause precipitation as larger particles)
Guaifed (slow release)
Guaifed-PD (slow release)
Humibid DM (slow release)
Humibid DM Sprinkle (slow release)
Humibid L.A. (slow release)
Humibid Sprinkle (slow release)
Hydergine LC (liquid within a capsule)
Hydergine Sublingual (sublingual)
Hytakerol (liquid filled)

Drugs that mustn't be crushed or dissolved (continued)

Iberet (slow release)
Iberet-500 (slow release)
Ilotycin (enteric coated)
Inderal LA (slow release)
Inderide LA (slow release)
Indocin SR (slow release)
Ionamin (slow release)
Isoclor Timesules (slow release)
Isoptin SR (slow release)
Isordil Sublingual (sublingual)
Isordil Tembids (slow release)
Isosorbide Dinitrate SR (slow release)
Isosorbide Dinitrate Sublingual (sublingual)
Isuprel Glossets (sublingual)
Kaon Cl (slow release)
Klor-Con (slow release)
Klotrix (slow release)
K-Tab (slow release)
K + 10 (slow release)
Levsinex Timecaps (slow release)
Lithobid (slow release)
Meprospan (slow release)
Mestinon Timespans (slow release)
MI-Cebrin (enteric coated)
MI-Cebrin T (enteric coated)
Micro-K (slow release)
Motrin (taste)
M S Contin (slow release)
Naldecon (slow release)
Nico-400 (slow release)
Nicobid (slow release)
Nitro-Bid (slow release)
Nitrocine Timecaps (slow release)
Nitroglyn (slow release)
Nitrong (sublingual)
Nitrostat (sublingual)
Noctec (liquid within a capsule)
Nolamine (slow release)
Nolex LA (slow release)
Norflex (slow release)
Norpace CR (slow release)
Novafed (slow release)
Novafed A (slow release)
Optilets-500 Filmtab (enteric coated)
Optilets-M-500 Filmtab (enteric coated)

Ornade Spansules (slow release)
Pabalate (enteric coated)
Pabalate-SF (enteric coated)
Pancrease (enteric coated)
Pancrease MT (enteric coated)
Papaverine Sustained Action (slow release)
Pathilon Sequels (slow release)
Pavabid Plateau Caps (slow release)
PBZ-SR (slow release)
Perdiem (wax coated)
Peritrate SA (slow release)
Permitil Chronotab (slow release)
Phazyme (slow release)
Phazyme 95 (slow release)
Phenergan (taste)
Phyllocontin (slow release)
Plendil (slow release)
Polaramine Repetabs (slow release)
Prelu-2 (slow release)
Prilosec (slow release)
Pro-Banthine (taste)
Procainamide HCl SR (slow release)
Procan SR (slow release)
Procardia (delays absorption)
Procardia XL (slow release)
Pronestyl-SR (slow release)
Proventil Repetabs (slow release)
Prozac (slow release)
Quadra Hist (slow release)
Quibron-T/SR (slow release)
Quinaglute Dura-tabs (slow release)
Quinalan Lanatabs (slow release)
Quinalan SR (slow release)
Quinidex Extentabs (slow release)
Respaire-SR (slow release)
Respbid (slow release)
Ritalin-SR (slow release)
Robimycin Robitab (enteric coated)
Rondec-TR (slow release)
Roxanol SR (slow release)
Ru-Tuss (slow release)
Ru-Tuss DE (slow release)
Sinemet CR (slow release)
Singlet (slow release)

Slo-Phyllin GG (slow release)
Slo-Phyllin Gyrocaps (slow release)
Slow-Fe (slow release)
Slow-K (slow release)
Slow-Mag (slow release)
Sorbitrate SA (slow release)
Sorbitrate Sublingual (sublingual)
Sparine (taste)
S-P-T (liquid gelatin suspension)
Sudafed 12 Hour (slow release)
Sustaire (slow release)
Tavist-D (multiple compressed tablet)
Tedral SA (slow release)
Teldrin (slow release)
Tepanil Ten-Tab (slow release)
Tessalon Perles (slow release)
Theobid (slow release)
Theobid Jr. (slow release)
Theochron (slow release)
Theoclear L.A. (slow release)
Theo-Dur (slow release)
Theo-Dur Sprinkle (slow release)
Theolair-SR (slow release)
Theo-Sav (slow release)
Theo-24 (slow release)
Theovent (slow release)
Theox (slow release)
Therapy Bayer (enteric coated)
Thorazine Spansule (slow release)
Toprol XL (slow release)
T-Phyl (slow release)
Trental (slow release)
Triaminic (slow release)
Triaminic-12 (slow release)
Trilafon Repetabs (slow release)
Triptone Caplets (slow release)
Tuss-LA (slow release)
Tuss-Ornade Spansules (slow release)
Uniphyl (slow release)
ULR-LA (slow release)
Valrelease (slow release)
Verelan (slow release)
Wellbutrin (anesthetizes mucous membrane)
Wyamycin-S (slow release)
Wygesic (taste)
ZORprin (slow release)
Zymase (enteric coated)

Adapted with permission from Mitchell, J.F., and Pawlicki, K.S. "Oral Dosage Forms That Should Not Be Crushed, 1992 Revision," *Hospital Pharmacy* 27(8):690-92, 695-99, August 1992.

GIVING DRUGS THROUGH TUBES

If your patient has a nasogastric (NG) tube in place, you may need to give medications through it if the tube isn't attached to a suctioning device. Or you may need to give medications through a gastrostomy tube or a gastrostomy button. Keep in mind that all medications instilled through a tube should be in liquid form. If necessary, you may crush and dissolve some solid medications before instillation. Just make sure that they're crushable.

To instill drugs through tubes, first collect the necessary equipment. You'll need the patient's medi-cation record, the prescribed medication, a towel or linen-saver pad, a stethoscope, gloves, tissues, a glass of water, and a 50- or 60-ml piston-type, catheter-tipped syringe.

To give a crushable tablet, obtain a mortar and pestle for crushing and a liquid to dissolve the med-ication in just before instillation.

To give medication through a gastrostomy button, obtain a feeding tube appropriate for that particular button.

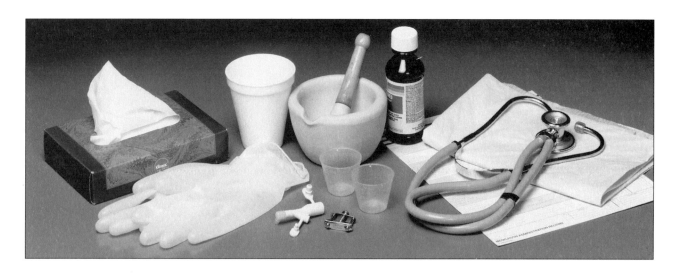

Giving a drug through an NG tube

To begin, place the patient in semi-Fowler's position. Wash your hands and put on gloves. To pro-tect the patient from spills, cover him with the towel or linen-saver pad. Next, remove the clamp from the NG tube and check the tube's position. To do this, insert the catheter-tipped syringe into the distal end of the tube, and aspi-rate a small amount of stomach contents. If stomach contents don't return to the syringe, place the diaphragm of your stethoscope over the patient's stomach. Then, listening with the stethoscope, in-still about 10 cc of air by the sy-ringe (as shown). If the tube is in the stomach, you'll hear a loud gurgle when you inject the air.

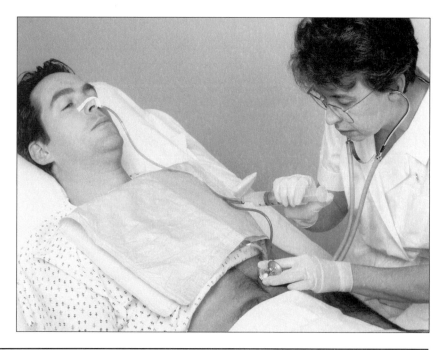

Once you've confirmed the tube's proper position, remove the syringe from the NG tube. Then remove the piston from the syringe. Insert the catheter tip into the NG tube port, making sure it fits snugly.

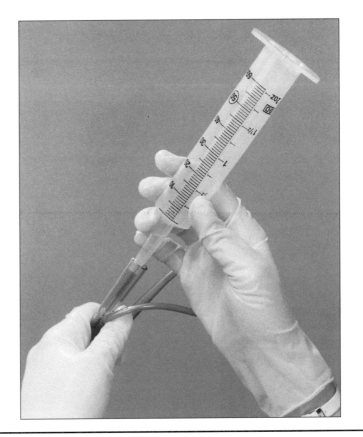

Hold the syringe attached to the NG tube upright, slightly above the level of the patient's nose.

Slowly pour the medication into the syringe, which acts as a funnel. Allow the medication to flow slowly through the tube. If the medication flows too fast, lower the syringe. If it flows too slowly, raise the syringe slightly. As the syringe empties, add the rest of the medication.

To prevent air from entering the stomach, avoid letting the syringe drain completely during administration.

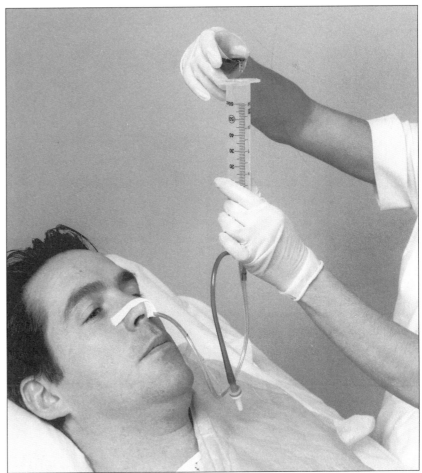

After giving all of the medication, pour 30 to 50 ml of water into the syringe. Let the water flow through the tube to rinse it and to ensure that all of the medication reaches the stomach.

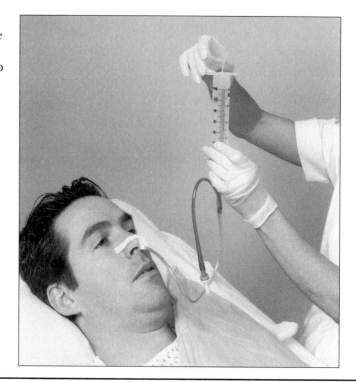

Next, clamp the tube and remove the syringe. Clean and store the equipment, or dispose of it, as appropriate.

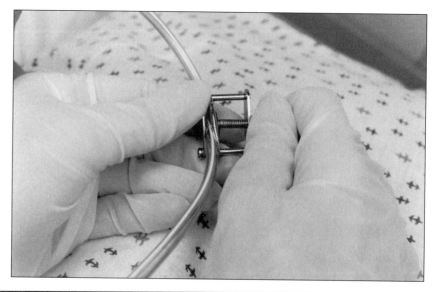

Have the patient remain in semi-Fowler's position, or allow him to lie on his side, for at least 30 minutes to prevent esophageal reflux.

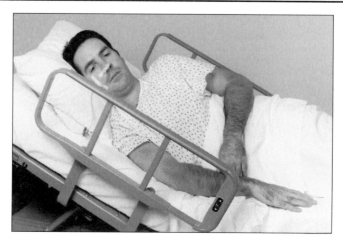

Giving a drug through a gastrostomy tube

To deliver a drug through a gastrostomy tube, prepare the medication as you would for NG tube delivery. Put on gloves. Remove the dressing covering the tube, if necessary, as well as the dressing or plug (as shown) at the distal tip of the tube.

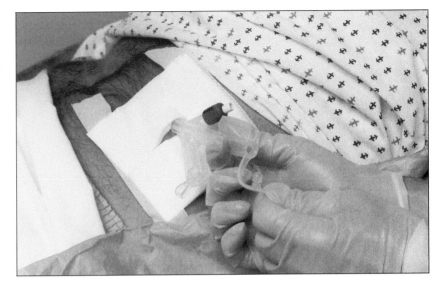

Remove the piston from the catheter-tipped syringe, and insert the catheter into the gastrostomy tube. Release the clamp on the tube and check the tube's patency by instilling about 10 ml of water. If the water flows freely, the tube is patent.

Then you can pour up to 30 ml of medication into the syringe (as shown). Regulate the flow rate by raising or lowering the syringe. After giving all of the medication, instill about 30 ml of water to rinse the tube.

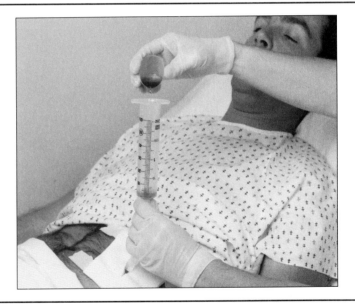

Remove the syringe from the tube and tighten the clamp. Replug the gastrostomy tube opening. Keep the patient in semi-Fowler's position for at least 30 minutes to prevent esophageal reflux.

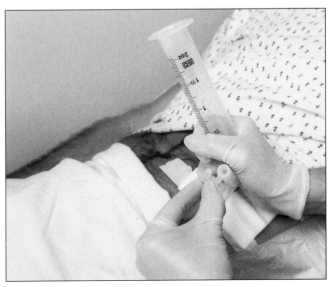

Giving a drug through a gastrostomy button

To instill a drug through a gastrostomy button, prepare the medication as you would for NG tube instillation. Also, obtain a feeding tube to fit the patient's kind of button.

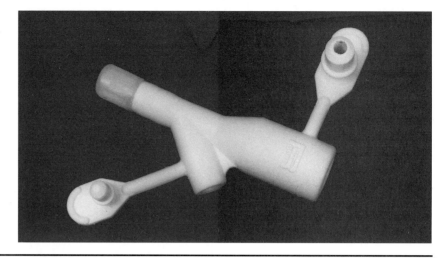

Put on gloves. Remove the safety plug and attach the feeding tube to the gastrostomy button. (The illustration clarifies how this attachment is made.)

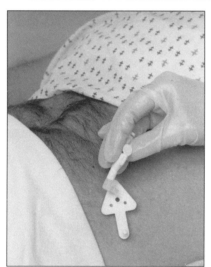

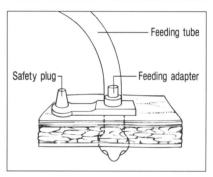

Remove the piston from the catheter-tipped syringe, and insert the catheter into the distal end of the tube. Check for patency, as you would for a gastrostomy tube. Then pour the prescribed medication into the syringe (as shown near right) and allow it to flow into the stomach.

After instilling all of the medication, pour 30 to 50 ml of water into the syringe and allow it to flow through the tube. When all of the water has been delivered, remove the feeding tube and replace the safety plug (as shown far right). Have the patient remain in semi-Fowler's position for at least 30 minutes to prevent esophageal reflux.

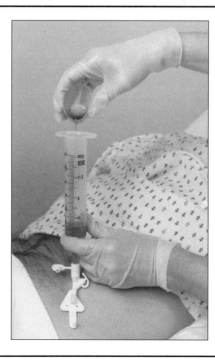

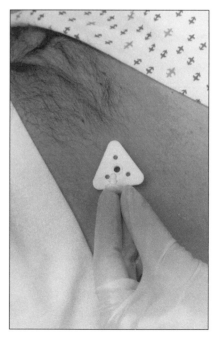

GIVING NASAL DRUGS

For the most part, nasal drugs produce local effects. Use drops to medicate a specific nasal area and sprays and aerosols to diffuse medication in the nasal passages. The most commonly administered nasal drugs are vasoconstrictors, which coat and shrink swollen mucous membranes. Other nasal drugs include local anesthetics, which promote patient comfort with procedures such as bronchoscopy, and corticosteroids, which reduce inflammation from allergies, infections, and nasal polyps. For best effect, deliver nose drops directly onto the mucous membranes. (See *Positioning the patient for nose drops*.)

Positioning the patient for nose drops

To ensure the maximum benefit of nasal medication, be sure to position the patient so that the drops don't flow into the pharynx.

To treat nasal congestion
To relieve an ordinary stuffy nose, apply drops to the nasal mucosa. The patient should be reclining or supine, with his head slightly tilted toward the affected side. Aim the dropper upward toward the patient's eye, rather than downward toward his ear.

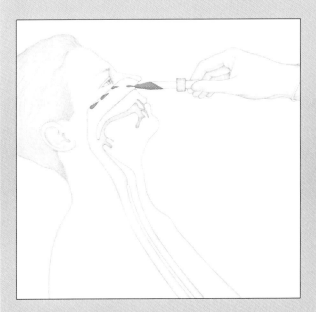

To treat the sinuses
To treat the ethmoid and sphenoid sinuses, position the patient on his back, with his neck hyperextended and his head tilted back over the edge of the bed. Support his head with one hand to prevent neck strain, as shown at the top of the next column.

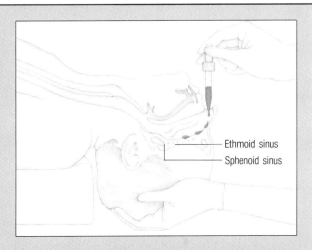

Ethmoid sinus
Sphenoid sinus

To treat the maxillary and frontal sinuses, have the patient lie on his back, with his head tilted toward the affected side and hanging over the edge of the bed. Ask him to turn his head sideways after he hyperextends his neck. Support his head with your hand to prevent neck strain.

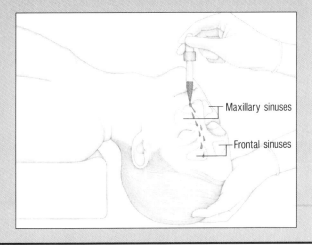

Maxillary sinuses
Frontal sinuses

Beverly A. Tscheschlog, RN, who contributed to this section, is a clinical consultant for Springhouse Corporation. The publisher also thanks *Village Pharmacy at Springhouse (Pa.)* for its help.

Giving nose drops to an adult

After verifying the medication order, gather the equipment you'll need, including the prescribed medication, the patient's medication record, an emesis basin, facial tissues, gloves, and a pillow (optional).

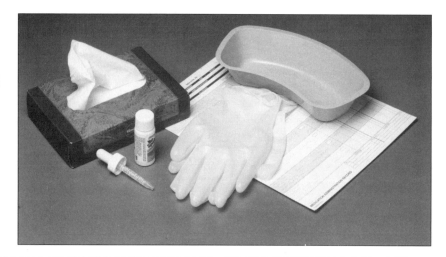

Check the patient's identity and explain the procedure to her. Position her as needed to ensure that the drops reach the intended site.

Wash your hands and put on gloves. Then uncap the nose drop bottle, and squeeze the bulb on the nose dropper to withdraw the prescribed dose from the bottle.

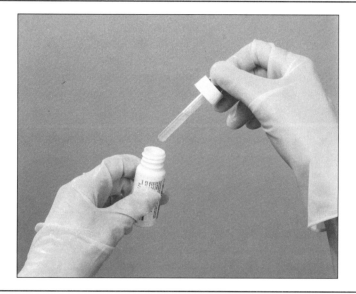

Push up gently on the tip of the patient's nose to open her nostril completely.

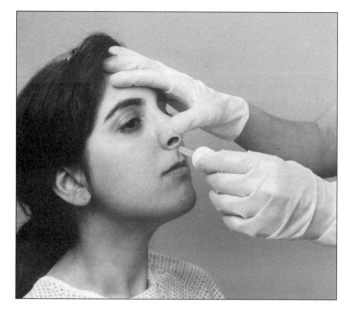

Place the dropper about ⅓″ (1 cm) inside the nostril. Slightly angle the tip of the dropper toward the inner corner of the patient's eye. Squeeze the dropper bulb to dispense the correct number of drops into each nostril.

▶ *Clinical tip:* To minimize the risk of contaminating the dropper, take care not to let it touch the patient's nose.

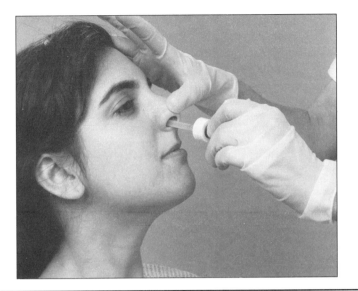

After you instill the prescribed number of drops, instruct the patient to keep her head tilted back for about 5 minutes. Encourage her to expectorate any medication that runs into her throat. Then document drug administration.

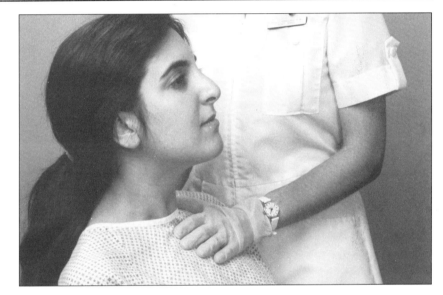

Stay with the patient. Encourage her to breathe through her mouth. If she coughs, help her to sit upright and gently pat her back. For several minutes, observe her closely for possible respiratory problems.

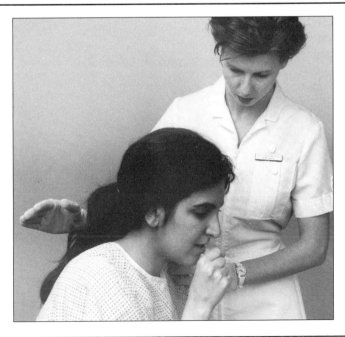

Giving nose drops to an infant or a child

To administer nasal medication to an infant, obtain the medication and warm it. Do this by holding the closed nose drop bottle under warm water. Then wash your hands and put on gloves. Position the infant on your arm so that her head tilts backward.

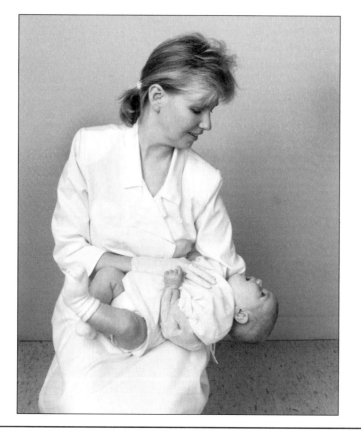

Draw up the medication by squeezing on the dropper's bulb until the correct dose fills the dropper. Open the infant's nostril, taking care also to support the head.

Instill the medication and keep the infant's head tilted back for 5 minutes. Observe for signs of aspiration. If the infant begins to cough, help her to an upright sitting position and gently pat her on the back until she clears her lungs. Then document drug administration.

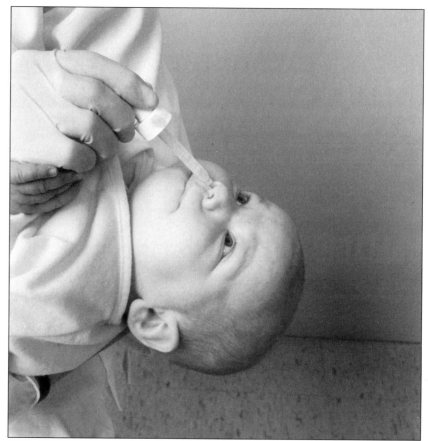

To give nose drops to a child who's too large to hold in your arms, you'll need a pillow. Have the child lie on his back, and place the pillow under his shoulders. Gently tilt his head back, supporting it between your forearm and body. Use your other arm to steady his position and, if necessary, to restrain his arms and hands. Instill the medication, and keep the child's head tilted back for about 5 minutes.

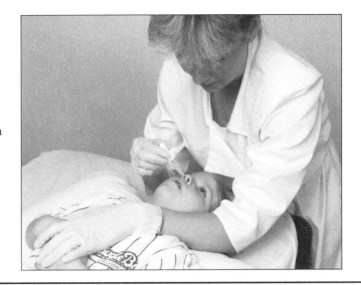

Delivering a nasal spray

Nasal sprays break medication into small particles and distribute it evenly over the mucous membranes. To begin administration, wash your hands and gather the needed equipment, including the prescribed medication in an atomizer, the patient's medication record, an emesis basin, facial tissues, gloves, and a pillow (optional).

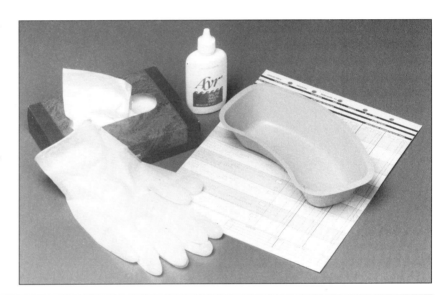

Put on gloves and have the patient sit straight with her head upright.
▶ *Clinical tip:* With many patients, you'll find administration to be more effective if you explain the procedure and have the patient perform it while you supervise.

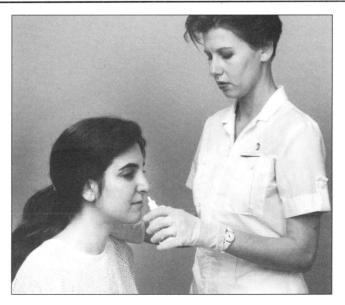

Occlude one nostril with your index finger. Place the tip of the atomizer about ½″ (1 cm) inside the patient's open nostril. Position the tip straight up the nose toward the inner corner of the eye. Depending on the drug, have the patient hold her breath or inhale. Then squeeze the atomizer once—quickly and firmly—just enough for the medication to coat the inside of the nose. Excessive force may propel the medication into the patient's sinuses and cause a headache. Repeat the procedure in the other nostril, as ordered.

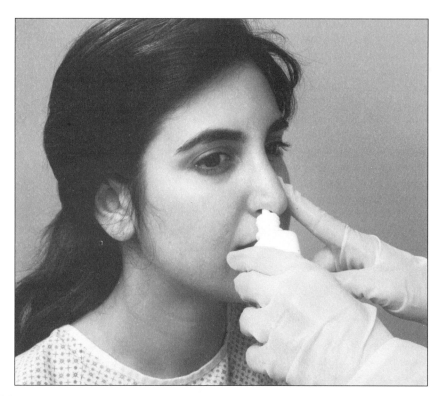

Tell the patient to keep her head tilted back for several minutes so that the medication has time to work. Instruct her not to blow her nose during that time.

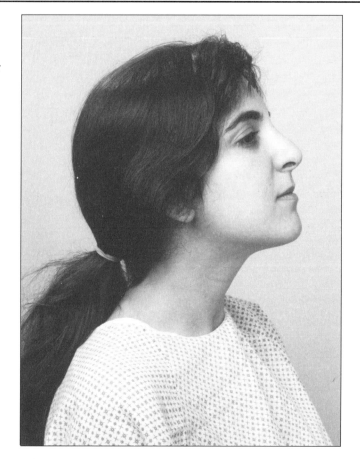

GIVING SUBLINGUAL, BUCCAL, AND TRANSLINGUAL DRUGS

When the doctor prescribes a drug in sublingual, buccal, or translingual form, he does so to prevent its destruction or transformation in the stomach or small intestine. Sublingual, buccal, and translingual drugs act quickly because the oral mucosa's thin epithelium and abundant vasculature promote the drug's direct absorption into the bloodstream.

Drugs given sublingually include ergotamine tartrate, erythrityl tetranitrate, isoproterenol hydrochloride, isosorbide dinitrate, and nitroglycerin. Drugs given buccally include erythrityl tetranitrate and methyltestosterone.

Advise the patient who's taking a drug sublingually or buccally not to smoke before the drug has dissolved. That's because nicotine's vasoconstrictive effects slow absorption.

Tell the patient taking nitroglycerin tablets to wet the tablet with saliva before putting it in his mouth. This speeds absorption.

Instruct the patient taking buccal tablets that are absorbed slowly (some may take up to 1 hour to be absorbed) not to eat or ingest liquids while the tablet is in the mouth. Otherwise, he might swallow the tablet.

Some sublingual drugs—erythrityl tetranitrate, for example—may cause a tingling sensation under the tongue. If the patient finds this bothersome, placing the drug in the buccal pouch instead may help.

▶ *Clinical tip:* When you give a sublingual or buccal drug, observe your patient to ensure that he doesn't swallow the medication. Also, inspect his oral mucosa for irritation caused by continuous buccal administration. And remember to alternate drug placement sites and to administer sublingual or buccal tablets *after* you give all other oral drugs.

Translingual drugs, which are sprayed onto the tongue, include nitrate preparations for patients with chronic angina. They may be administered prophylactically before stressful activities or at the onset of an attack.

Advise the patient who's using a translingual spray to familiarize himself with the position of the spray orifice. This orifice can be identified by the finger rest on top of the valve. Learning to handle the container will be particularly helpful for using the medication at night.

To give these medications, you'll need the patient's medication record, the ordered medication, and a medication cup. You'll also need gloves. To begin, match the drug order with the patient's medication record, and confirm the patient's identity. Do this by asking his name and checking his identification bracelet.

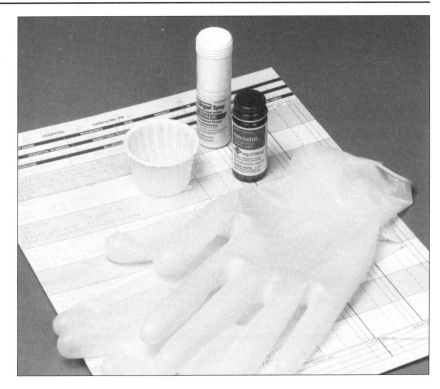

Wash your hands and put on gloves. Remove the tablet from the patient's medication drawer and place it in the medication cup. To give the tablet sublingually, place it under the patient's tongue. Instruct the patient to keep the medication in place until it dissolves completely and not to chew the tablet or drink any water or smoke for 1 hour.

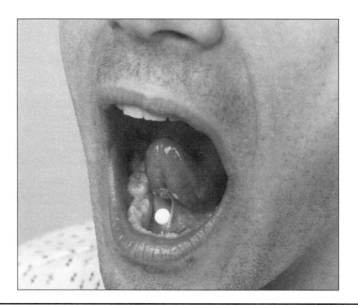

To administer a buccal medication, place the tablet between the patient's cheek and teeth. Instruct him to close his mouth and hold the tablet against his cheek until the tablet is absorbed.

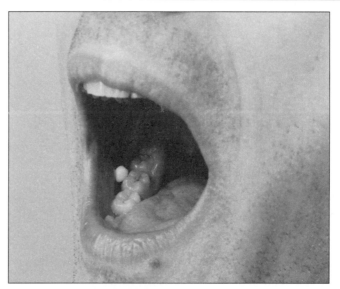

To administer a translingual spray, tell the patient to hold the medication canister vertically, with the valve head uppermost and the spray orifice as close to his mouth as possible. Instruct him to spray the dose onto the tongue by pressing the button firmly.

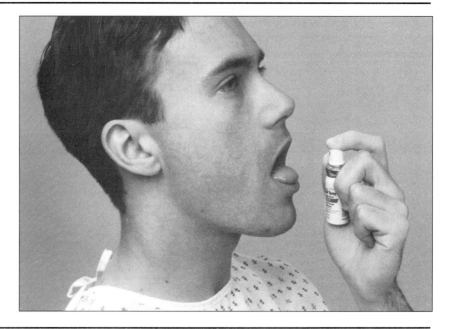

APPLYING TOPICAL DRUGS

Applied directly to the skin, topical drugs include creams, pastes, ointments, shampoos, lotions, sprays, powders, and assorted medicated dressings.

The body absorbs topical drugs through the epidermis and dermis. The extent of absorption depends on the area's vascularity. Except for nitroglycerin and certain hormones, topical drugs are used mostly to achieve local effects.

Different topical drug forms have distinct properties, making some more suitable than others for certain disorders or for particular skin areas, such as the scalp and face. Ointments, for instance, have a fatty base, making them an ideal form for antimicrobial and antiseptic drugs. (See *Guide to selected topical drug forms.*)

Another drug form tailored to a specific therapeutic aim is the medicated shampoo, including keratolytic and cytostatic agents, coal tar preparations, and lindane (gamma benzene hexachloride) solutions used to treat dandruff, psoriasis, and head lice, respectively. These products are contraindicated in patients with broken or abraded skin.

To prevent skin irritation from accumulated medication, don't apply a topical drug without first removing the residue from previous applications. Additional considerations include the following:
• Wear gloves to prevent drug absorption by your own skin and to avoid cross-contamination.
• Don't apply ointments to mucous membranes as liberally as you would to skin. That's because mucous membranes are usually moist and absorb ointment more quickly than skin does.
• Avoid applying too much ointment to any skin area. It may cause irritation and discomfort, stain clothing and bedding, and make removal difficult.
• Never apply ointments to the eyelids or ear canal unless ordered. The substance may congeal and occlude the tear duct or ear canal.

Guide to selected topical drug forms

Use this guide to understand the effects of different topical drug forms and to help plan nursing care.

DRUG FORM	EFFECTS	NURSING CONSIDERATIONS
Cream An oil-in-water semisolid emulsion	• Acts as a barrier	• Apply cream to clean, dry skin. • Thoroughly massage cream into the skin. • After application, observe skin for irritation.
Paste A stiff mixture of powder and ointment	• Provides a uniform coating of medication • Reduces and repels moisture	• Apply paste to clean, dry skin. • Cover the medicated area to increase absorption and to protect the patient's clothing and bed linen.
Ointment Oil and water in a semisolid suspension	• Retains body heat • Provides prolonged contact with medication	• To increase absorption, warm the patient's skin with heat packs or a warm bath before applying. • Apply ointment to clean, dry skin. • As directed, apply a thin layer of ointment to the patient's skin and rub it in well. • Use care when applying ointment to draining wounds.
Lotion A suspension of insoluble powder in water or an emulsion without powder	• Creates sensation of dryness • Leaves uniform and powdery surface film • Soothes, cools, and protects the skin	• Shake container well before using. • To increase absorption in certain skin conditions, warm the patient's skin with heat packs or a bath before applying. • Apply lotion to clean, dry skin. • Thoroughly massage lotion into the skin. • After application, observe skin for irritation.
Powder An inert chemical that may contain medication	• Promotes skin drying • Reduces moisture, maceration, and friction	• Apply powder to clean, dry skin. • To keep the patient from inhaling powder, instruct him to turn his head to the side during application. • If you're applying powder to the patient's face or neck, give him a cloth or a piece of gauze to mask his mouth. Direct him to exhale as you apply the powder.

Applying cream, paste, or ointment

Assemble the required equipment, including the prescribed medication, sterile tongue blades, gloves, sterile 4" × 4" gauze pads, a linen-saver pad or towel, and optional items (such as a transparent semipermeable dressing and adhesive tape) as needed.

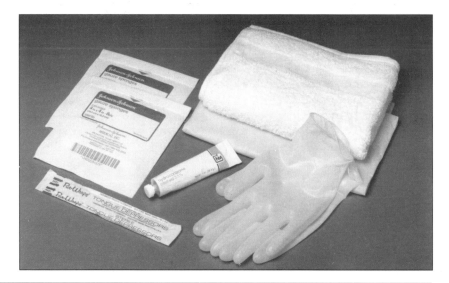

Verify the order on the patient's medication record, explain the procedure, and provide privacy. Wash your hands to prevent cross-contamination, and put on gloves. Help the patient into a comfortable position that provides access to the treatment area.

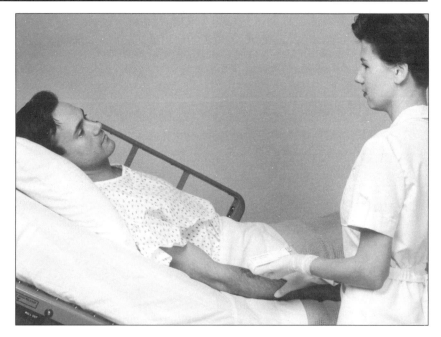

Expose the treatment area and place a linen-saver pad or towel under it, as shown. Make sure that the skin or mucous membrane is intact (unless the medication is for a skin lesion, such as an ulcer). If necessary, clean the area of debris by removing crusts, epidermal scales, and old medication. Change your gloves if they become soiled or if you're cleaning debris from the area.

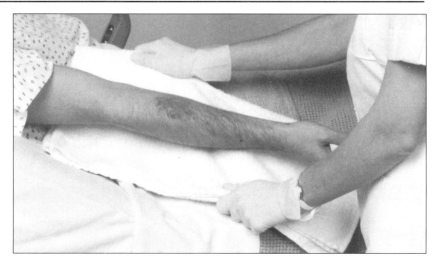

Open the medication container. Place the lid or cap upside down to protect the inside surface from contamination.

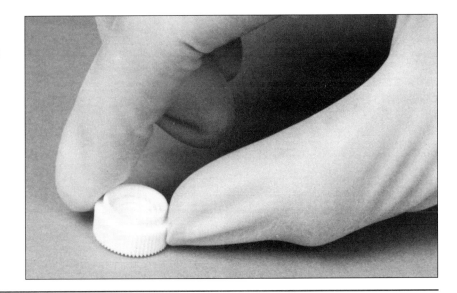

Remove a tongue blade from its sterile wrapper, and cover one end with medication from the tube or jar (near right). Transfer the medication from the tongue blade to your gloved hand (far right).

▶ *Clinical tip:* To prevent contamination, use a new tongue blade each time you take medication from the container.

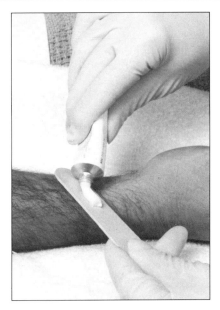 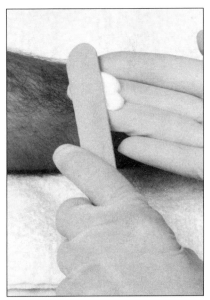

Apply the medication to the treatment area, using long, smooth strokes in the direction of hair growth. This prevents you from forcing medication into hair follicles, which can cause irritation and lead to folliculitis.

▶ *Clinical tip:* When applying topical medications, avoid excessive pressure, which could abrade the skin.

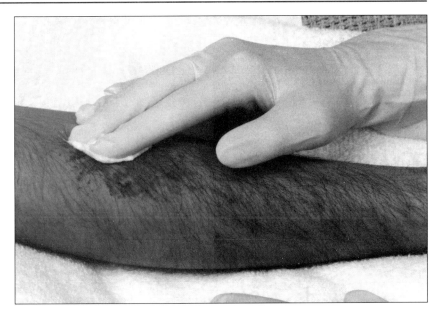

Removing ointment

Like oil and water, ointment and water don't mix. To remove ointment from your patient's skin, you'll need a solvent, such as cottonseed oil, and sterile 4″ × 4″ gauze pads. Saturate a 4″ × 4″ gauze pad with the cottonseed oil.

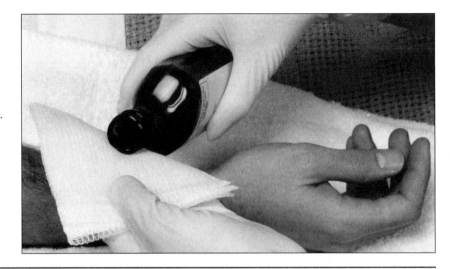

Use this pad to swab the ointment gently from the patient's skin (as shown). Remove any excess cottonseed oil by gently wiping the area with a clean sterile gauze pad. Don't wipe too hard, though, or you could irritate the skin.

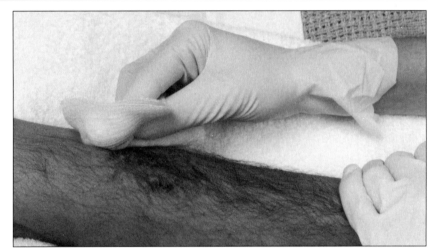

Applying a spray or a powder

Gather the equipment that you'll need, including the prescribed medicated spray or powder and towels or linen-saver pads, as needed. Before applying a spray, shake the medication container (near right). Hold the container 6″ to 12″ (15 to 30 cm) from the skin or as directed by the product label and begin spraying (far right).

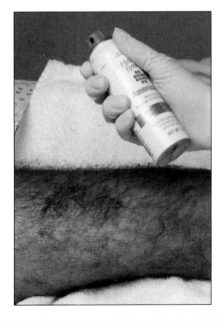
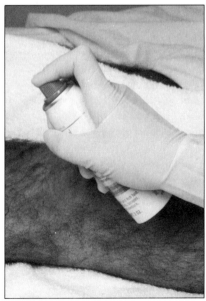

To apply a powder, first dry the skin surface, making sure that you spread and dry any skin folds where moisture collects.

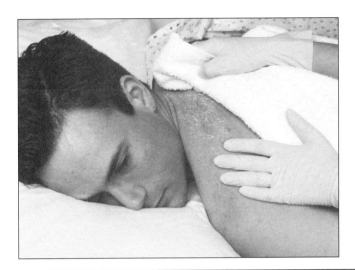

Apply a thin layer of powder over the treatment area.
▶ ***Clinical tip:*** To protect the patient from inhaling any airborne powder unnecessarily, shake the powder onto your hand and then apply it gently to his skin.

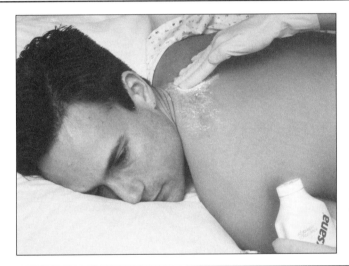

Applying a topical drug to the scalp

Whether you're applying a medicated lotion, cream, or shampoo to the patient's scalp, you'll proceed similarly, but you'll work shampoo into a lather, which you won't do with other scalp medications. First assemble your equipment: medication, shampoo, or both as needed; towels; linen-saver pads; and a comb. Then wash the patient's hair. After drying his hair and scalp with a towel, comb out any tangles.

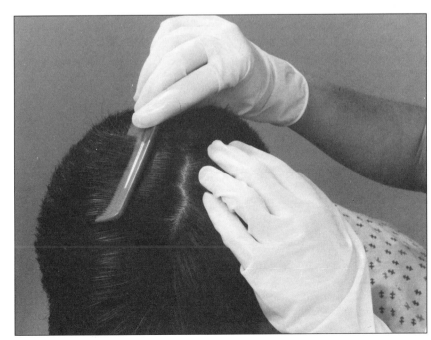

Using your fingertips, apply medication to the scalp, starting at the point where the hair parts naturally. Spread the medication evenly.

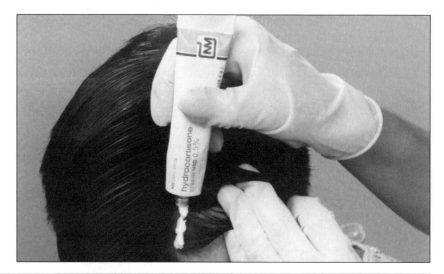

Continue applying the medication every ½" (1 cm), following instructions on the product label. If directed, massage the medication into the scalp, taking care not to use your fingernails. Repeat as instructed.

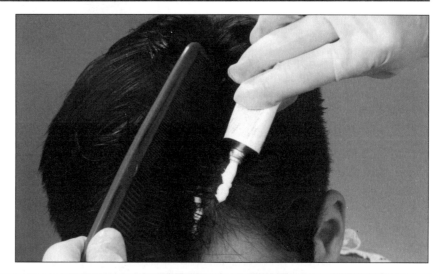

If you're using a medicated shampoo, shake the bottle of shampoo well to mix the solution evenly. Wet the patient's hair thoroughly, and wring out excess water. Part the hair and apply the shampoo, working it into a lather and adding water as needed. Lather the scalp and hair for as long as instructed. Then rinse the hair.

▶ *Clinical tip:* Read the label carefully to make sure that you apply the shampoo as directed and understand corrective actions to take in case of an accident. (For instance, some shampoos contain selenium sulfide, which is extremely toxic if ingested. Other products can harm the eyes and need to be flushed from the eyes promptly with water.)

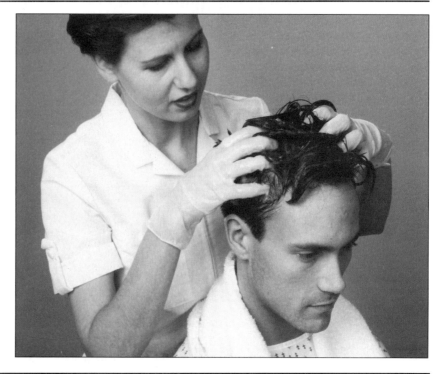

After rinsing the medicated shampoo from the patient's hair, remove excess moisture with a towel. Then comb or brush the hair.

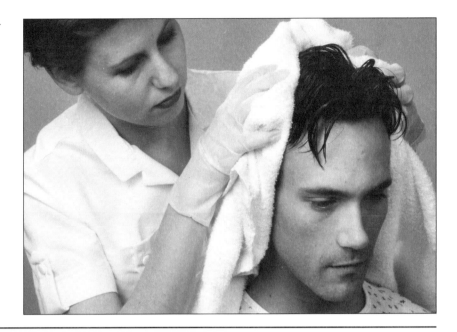

Applying a drug to the face

To apply a drug to your patient's face, first assemble soap and water, cotton-tipped applicators, sterile 4″ × 4″ gauze pads, the prescribed medication, towels, and a washcloth. Then clean the patient's face with mild soap and water to remove any previous medication residue or exudate.

To apply medication to small areas (forehead, chin, or under eyes), use a cotton-tipped applicator.

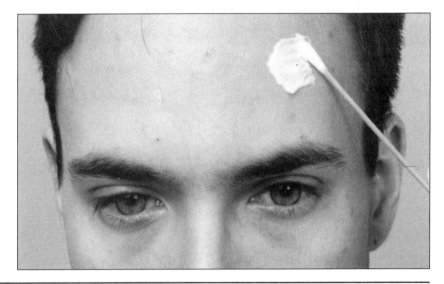

To apply medication to large facial areas, use a 4″ × 4″ gauze pad.

▶ *Clinical tip:* Always begin by applying the medication to the patient's forehead. Then spread it down each side of the face to the jaw. Stroke in one direction only.

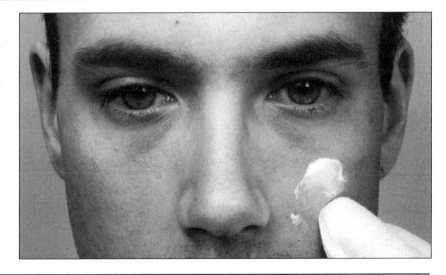

Applying the right dressing

You may need to apply a permeable, a semipermeable, or an occlusive medicated dressing to treat skin problems—especially when the patient can't tolerate a bath, when the skin problem affects an area that can't be soaked, or when the skin needs long-term treatment and protection.

A permeable dressing allows air to reach the wound. A semipermeable dressing allows oxygen to reach the wound. An occlusive dressing, which is impermeable to oxygen, reduces wound pain, speeds reepithelialization, and stimulates debridement and healing.

Use the following chart as a guide to these different dressings. And be sure to apply the dressing correctly. Incorrect application can macerate the skin and stain clothing and bed linen.

DRESSING TYPE	USES	BENEFITS	NURSING CONSIDERATIONS
Open, wet dressing (permeable)	• Acute inflammatory skin conditions, erosions, ulcers • Skin lesions with oozing exudate	• Delivers medication • Softens and heals the skin • Absorbs pus and exudate • Decreases blood flow to inflamed areas • Helps promote drainage • Protects site from contamination	• Apply this medication-soaked dressing to the skin, and leave the dressing uncovered. Remoisten the dressing when the water in the medication evaporates. • You may use an open, wet dressing, for example, to apply a solution of water and aluminum sulfate (such as Domeboro powder).
Closed, wet dressing (occlusive)	• Cellulitis • Erysipelas • Psoriasis • Lichen simplex chronicus • Eczema	• Delivers medication • Softens and heals the skin • Increases effectiveness of medication • Absorbs pus and exudate • Increases blood flow to inflamed areas • Protects site from contamination	• Apply this medication-soaked dressing to the skin, and cover the dressing with an occlusive or insulative bandage. Covering the dressing this way helps to prevent water evaporation and heat loss. • You may use an occlusive dressing, for example, to apply desoximetasone (Topicort) and an insulative dressing to apply boric acid solution.
Wet-to-dry dressing (permeable)	• Wound debridement	• Delivers medication • Softens the skin • Absorbs pus, exudate, debris, and eschar	• Apply this dressing in the same way as you would the open, wet dressing. However, when the water evaporates, remove the dressing; don't remoisten it. • You may use a wet-to-dry dressing, for example, to apply sodium hypochlorite (Dakin's solution).
Dry dressing (semipermeable)	• Neurodermatitis • Stasis dermatitis	• Protects skin from abrasion • Protects site from contamination	• Apply this ordinary gauze pad to the skin. • You may use a dry dressing, for example, with a debriding agent such as collagenase (Collagenase ABC).

GIVING TRANSDERMAL DRUGS

Through a measured dose of ointment or an adhesive patch applied to the skin, transdermal drugs deliver a constant, controlled amount of medication to the bloodstream, thereby achieving a prolonged effect. Typical drugs currently available in transdermal form include nitroglycerin (to control angina), scopolamine (to treat motion sickness), estradiol (to provide hormone replacement after menopause), clonidine (to treat hypertension), and fentanyl (to control chronic pain).

Differences in transdermal forms usually reflect drug delivery times. For example, transdermal nitroglycerin ointment dilates coronary vessels for up to 4 hours, whereas a nitroglycerin patch (or disk) produces the same effect for as long as 24 hours. In patch form, scopolamine can relieve motion sickness for as long as 72 hours; estradiol lasts for up to 1 week; clonidine, for 24 hours; and fentanyl, up to 72 hours. (See *Understanding transdermal disks*.)

NURSING CONSIDERATIONS

When administering transdermal medications, keep these points in mind:
• Apply the drug at regular and appropriate times to ensure a continuous effect.
• Avoid applying the drug if the patient has skin allergies or has experienced skin reactions to the drug. Don't apply transdermal drugs to broken or irritated skin because the drug may increase irritation.
• Select a smooth application site. Avoid applying a transdermal drug to scarred or calloused skin because this may impair absorption.
• Review drug-specific precautions. For example, before reapplying nitroglycerin ointment, remove the plastic wrap, application strip, and any drug residue from the previous application site. When applying a scopolamine patch, instruct the patient not to drive or operate machinery until he's accustomed to his own response to the drug. Also, warn a patient using clonidine patches to check with his doctor before using any nonprescription cough preparations because they may counteract the effects of the drug.
• Inform the patient about possible adverse effects from transdermal drug delivery, such as skin irritation (pruritus or a rash). Explain other adverse effects as appropriate. For example, transdermal nitroglycerin medications may cause headaches and, in elderly patients, postural hypotension. Scopolamine has various adverse effects, but dry mouth and drowsiness are the most common. Transdermal estradiol increases the risk of endometrial cancer, thromboembolic disease, and birth defects. In addition, clonidine may cause severe rebound hypertension, especially if withdrawn suddenly.

Understanding transdermal disks

Transdermal drug disks consist of several layers.
• The adhesive layer closest to the patient's skin holds a small amount of the drug, which is absorbed through the skin and into the bloodstream.
• Membranelike, the next layer controls release of the drug from the disk core.
• The third layer (the drug reservoir) contains the main dose of the drug.
• The outermost layer consists of an aluminized polyester barrier that holds the drug in the disk.

   Note: The dots in the illustration at right represent drug absorption.

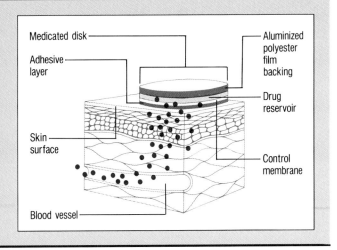

Beverly Tscheschlog, RN, a clinical consultant, contributed to this section. The publisher thanks the following organizations for their help: *Doylestown (Pa.) Hospital; Hill-Rom*, Batesville, Ind.; and *Village Pharmacy at Springhouse (Pa.)*

Applying transdermal drugs

Obtain the prescribed medication (disk, patch, or ointment), an application strip or measuring paper (for nitroglycerin ointment), and a semipermeable dressing or plastic wrap (optional for nitroglycerin ointment). Gloves are optional. Depending on the drug used, you may need a washcloth, soap and water, a towel, and adhesive tape. Verify the order on the patient's medication record. Then explain the procedure and provide privacy. Wash your hands and, if necessary, put on gloves.

▶ *Clinical tip:* Wear gloves to apply ointment so that your hands don't absorb the drug.

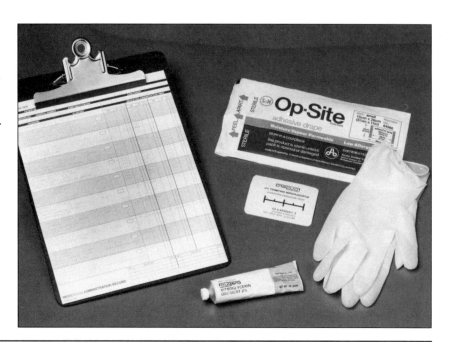

Applying transdermal ointment

Choose the application site—usually a dry, hairless spot on the patient's chest or arm. To promote absorption, wash the site with soap and warm water. If the patient has a previously applied medication strip, remove it and wash this area to remove any drug residue. Dry the application site thoroughly.

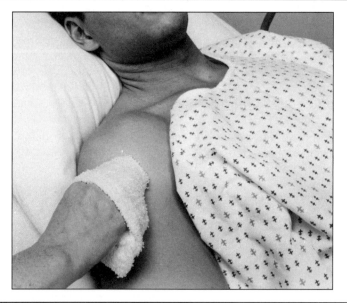

Squeeze the prescribed amount of ointment onto the application strip or measuring paper. Don't let any of the drug touch your skin.

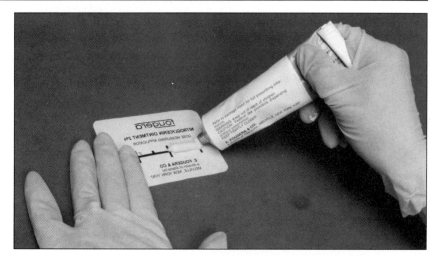

Apply the strip, drug side down, directly to the skin. Maneuver the strip slightly to spread a thin layer of the ointment over a 3″ (8-cm) area, but don't rub the ointment into the skin.

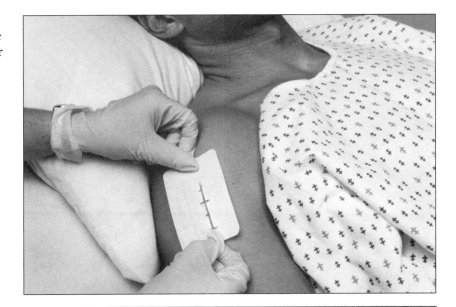

Secure the application strip to the skin by covering it with a semipermeable dressing or, if applying nitroglycerin ointment, the plastic wrap. Tape the plastic wrap in place.

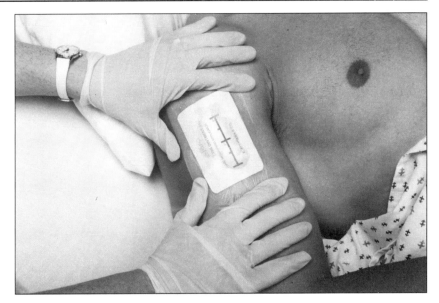

If required by your hospital policy, label the strip with the date, time, and your initials (as shown). If you didn't wear gloves, wash your hands immediately to avoid absorbing the drug. Instruct the patient to keep the area around the patch as dry as possible.

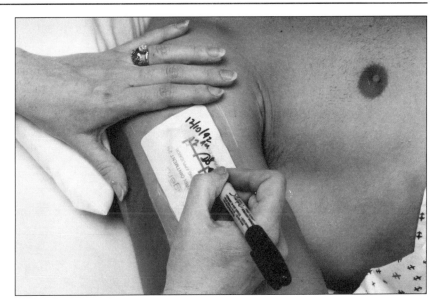

Applying a transdermal patch

Choose a dry, hairless application site. If necessary, clip any hair from the site, but don't shave the area. The most commonly used sites include the upper arm, chest, back, and behind the ear. Clean the application site with soap and warm water. Dry thoroughly. Open the drug package and remove the patch.

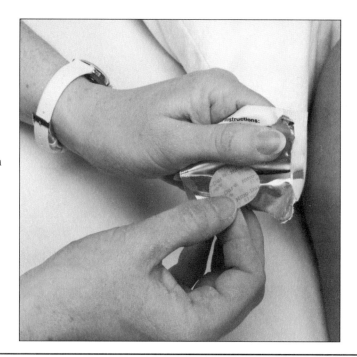

Without touching the adhesive surface, remove the clear plastic backing.

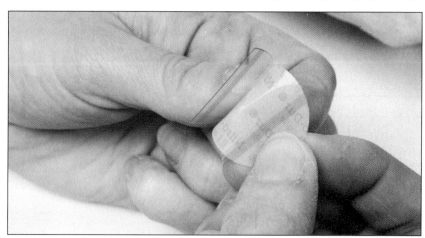

Without touching the patch's adhesive layer, apply the patch to the application site (as shown). If required by your hospital policy, label the site with the date, time, and your initials.

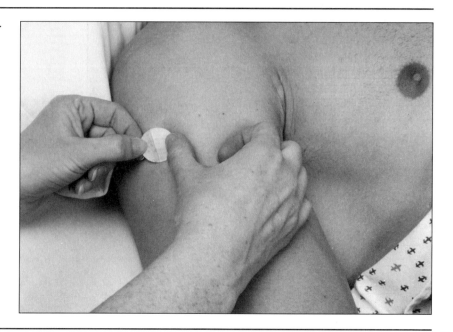

GIVING RECTAL DRUGS

Medication may be administered rectally to a patient who's unconscious, vomiting, or otherwise unable to swallow. Because rectal administration bypasses the upper GI tract, medications aren't destroyed in the stomach or small intestine by digestive enzymes. Nor do they irritate the upper GI tract, as some oral medications can. What's more, rectally administered medications bypass the portal system, thereby avoiding biotransformation in the liver.

But rectal drugs have some disadvantages. For instance, the procedure for administration may cause the patient discomfort or embarrassment. Also, the drug may be incompletely absorbed, especially if the patient can't retain it or if the rectum contains fecal matter. If absorption is incomplete, the patient may need a higher dose than he would if he were to take the same drug in oral form.

Suppositories, ointments, and medicated enemas are the most commonly given forms of rectal medication (see *Guide to rectal drug forms*).

NURSING CONSIDERATIONS

When administering medications rectally, keep the following tips in mind:
• Consider the patient's eating schedule before giving a medication to relieve constipation. That's because eating and drinking stimulate peristalsis. For the best effect, administer a suppository about 30 minutes before mealtime to soften the feces in the rectum and ease defecation. Also administer a retention suppository or enema between meals and after the patient empties his bladder and rectum.
• Before giving a retention enema, check the patient's elimination pattern. For example, a constipated patient may need a cleansing enema to prevent rectal feces from interfering with drug absorption. A patient with a fecal impaction may need the drug delivered by another route. Also, a patient with diarrhea may be unable to retain the enema solution for the prescribed time.
• Because inserting a rectal suppository or an enema tube usually stimulates the vagus nerve, rectal drug administration is contraindicated in patients with cardiac arrhythmias or myocardial infarction. You also may need to avoid it in patients who've had recent rectal, colon, or prostate surgery to minimize the risk of local trauma.
• Do not administer a rectal medication (or laxative) to a patient with undiagnosed abdominal pain. If the pain results from appendicitis, drug-induced peristaltic action could rupture the appendix.
• Before administering any rectal medication, inspect the patient's rectum. If the tissues are inflamed, the drug could aggravate the condition.

Guide to rectal drug forms

DRUG FORM	LOCAL USES	SYSTEMIC USES
Suppository Supplying a solid drug in a firm base, such as cocoa butter, suppositories melt at body temperature. These drugs are molded in cylindrical shapes usually about 1½" (4 cm) long (smaller for infants and children). Before using, keep suppositories refrigerated to prevent softening and possible decreased drug effectiveness.	• Relieves local pain and irritation • Promotes astringent action • Controls local itching • Reduces inflammation • Stimulates defecation • Lubricates and cleans • Relieves colic and gas	• Reduces pain and discomfort • Relieves nausea and vomiting • Reduces fever • Provides bronchodilation • Produces sedation • Promotes serenity and relaxation
Ointment This semisolid drug formulation may be applied externally to the anus or internally to the rectum.	• Reduces fever • Promotes astringent action • Relieves pain • Reduces inflammation • Kills bacteria	• None
Enema This is a liquid given rectally for retention (for at least 30 minutes or until absorbed, or for at least 10 minutes and then expelled). *Note:* Enemas given to clean the lower bowel are not medicated.	• Destroys parasites • Promotes astringent action • Stimulates defecation • Lubricates and cleans • Kills bacteria • Reduces inflammation	• Reduces fever • Promotes sedation • Anesthetizes • Supplies nutrition and hydration

Inserting a suppository

To administer a rectal suppository, you'll need the prescribed suppository, the patient's medication record and chart, several 4″ × 4″ gauze pads, gloves, a linen-saver pad, water-soluble lubricant, and, if indicated, a bedpan.

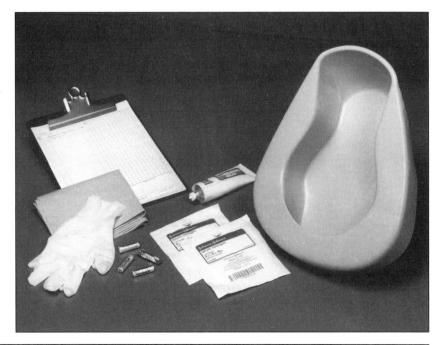

If the suppository softens too much for easy insertion, hold it (in its wrapper) under cold running water to harden it again.

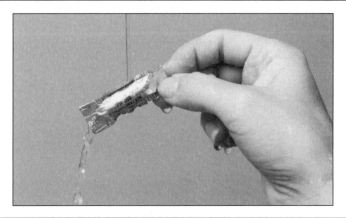

Match the patient's medication record with the doctor's order and confirm the patient's identity. Explain the procedure and its purpose to the patient. Provide privacy. Place the patient on the left side in Sims' position. Cover him with the bedcovers, exposing only the buttocks. Then place a linen-saver pad under the buttocks to protect the bedding.

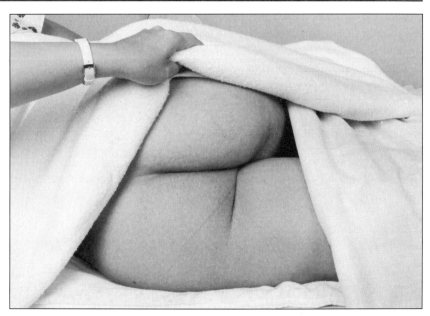

Put on gloves, and remove the suppository from its wrapper. Apply a water-soluble lubricant.

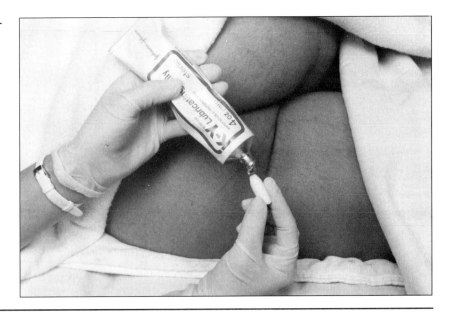

Using your nondominant hand, lift the patient's upper buttock to expose the anus.

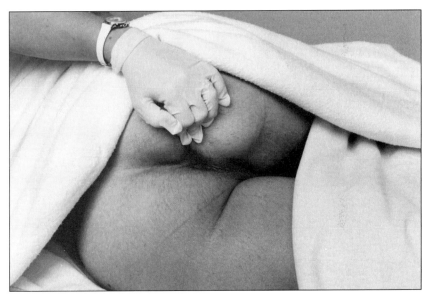

Instruct the patient to take several deep breaths through his mouth to relax the anal sphincter and reduce anxiety or discomfort during insertion. Then, using your dominant hand, insert the suppository—tapered end first—into the rectum. Use your index finger to direct the suppository along the rectal wall toward the umbilicus. Continue to advance it about 3″ (8 cm), or about the length of your finger, until it passes the patient's internal anal sphincter.

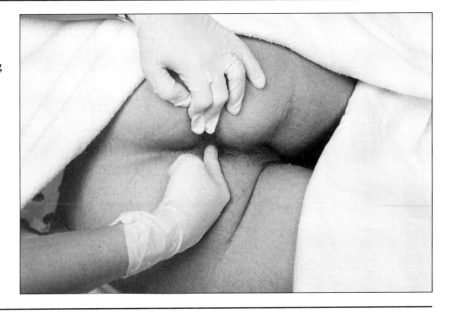

Ensure the patient's comfort. Encourage him to lie quietly and, if applicable, to retain the suppository for an appropriate time. A suppository administered to relieve constipation should be retained as long as possible (at least 20 minutes) to be effective. If necessary, press on the anus with a gauze pad (as shown) until the urge to defecate passes.

▶ *Clinical tip:* If the patient can't retain the suppository and pressing on the anus with a gauze pad fails to relieve the urge to defecate, place the patient on a bedpan. Inform him that the suppository may discolor his next bowel movement.

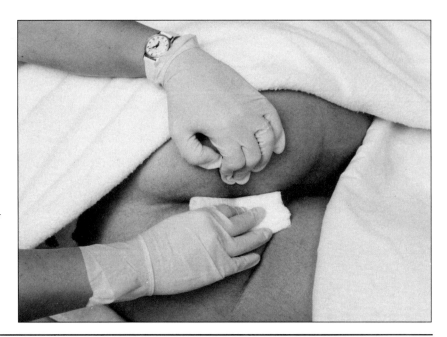

Applying rectal ointment externally

You'll need gloves, the prescribed ointment, and several 4″ × 4″ gauze pads. Put on gloves and squeeze a small amount of ointment on your finger.

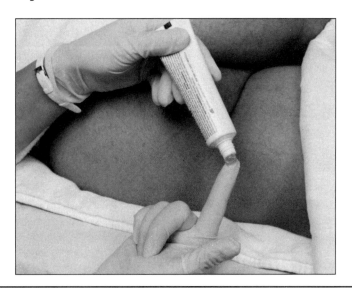

Spread the ointment over the anal area, using your gloved finger or a gauze pad.

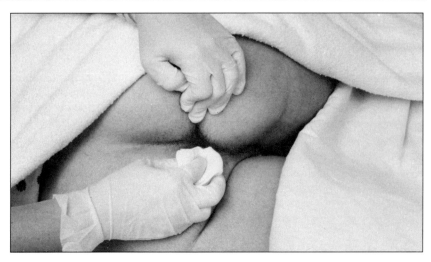

Applying rectal ointment internally

Gather the prescribed ointment, an applicator, several 4″ × 4″ gauze pads, and gloves. Put on the gloves. Remove the ointment tube's cap, and attach the applicator to the tube (near right).

Coat the applicator with water-soluble lubricant (far right). For internal administration, expect to use about 1″ (2.5 cm) of ointment. To judge the pressure needed to extract this amount, squeeze a small amount from the tube before you attach the applicator.

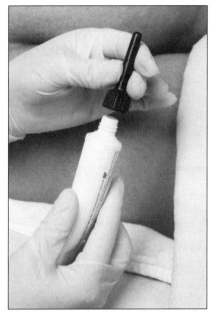 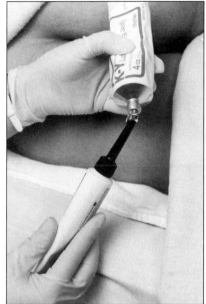

With your nondominant hand, lift the patient's upper buttock to expose the anus. Gently insert the applicator, directing it toward the umbilicus. Then slowly squeeze the tube to eject the medication.

▶ *Clinical tip:* Direct the patient to breathe deeply through his mouth to relax the anal sphincter and reduce anxiety or discomfort during insertion.

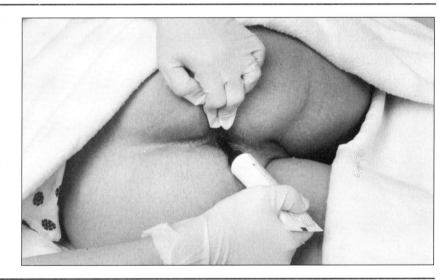

Withdraw the applicator and place a folded 4″ × 4″ gauze pad between the patient's buttocks (as shown) to absorb excess ointment. Remove the applicator from the tube and recap the tube. Clean the applicator with soap and water.

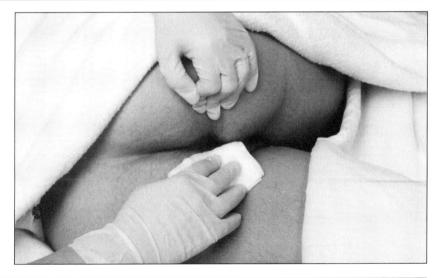

Instilling a retention enema

Administering drugs by enema involves having the patient retain a solution in the rectum or colon for 30 to 60 minutes. An adult requires 150 to 200 ml of fluid; a child over age 6, about 75 to 150 ml. (These amounts are smaller than those used for irrigating enemas.)

Obtain the prescribed solution (usually available in a premixed, commercially prepared container), a disposable enema kit or an enema bag assembly, gloves, 4″ × 4″ gauze pads, a bed pan, toilet paper, an emesis basin, a linen-saver pad, and water-soluble lubricant. You also may need an I.V. pole from which to hang the enema bag.

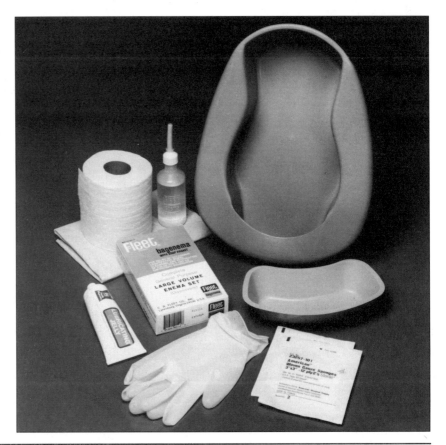

Explain the procedure to the patient. Stress the importance of retaining the solution until the medication is absorbed. To avoid stimulating peristalsis, have the patient empty his bladder and rectum before you begin.

Have the patient wear a gown, and provide privacy. Place a linen-saver pad under him and assist him into a left Sims' position. If he's uncomfortable in this position, reposition him on his right side or his back.

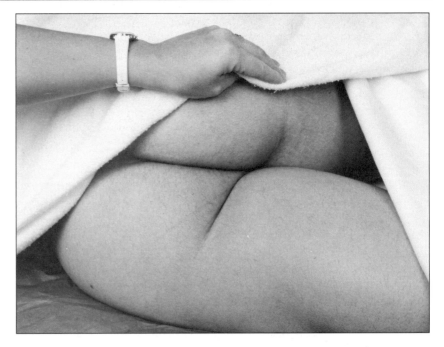

Administering a commercially prepared enema

Put on gloves and remove the cap from the rectal tube.

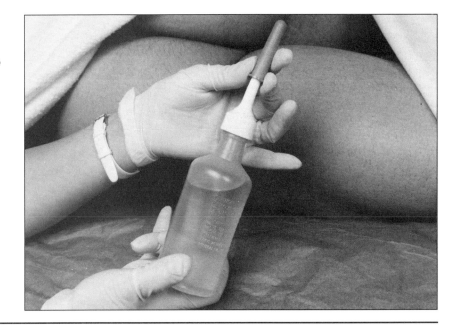

Check the amount of lubricant already on the rectal tube. If needed, squeeze additional water-soluble lubricant onto a 4″ × 4″ gauze pad, and dip the rectal tube's tip in the lubricant.

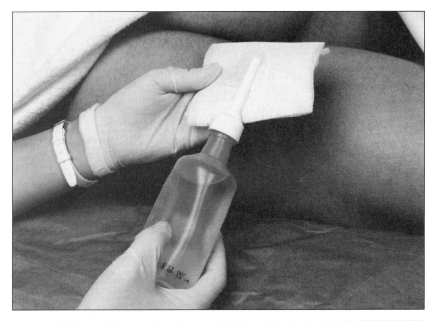

Gently squeeze the enema container to expel air.

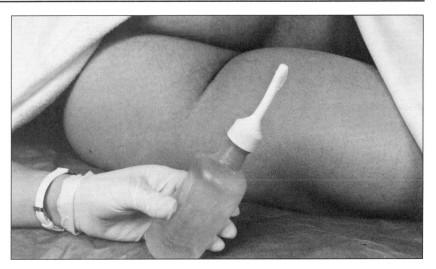

With your nondominant hand, lift the patient's upper buttock to expose the anus. Instruct the patient to take a deep breath. As the patient inhales, insert the rectal tube into the rectum, pointing the tube toward the umbilicus. For an adult, advance the tube 3″ to 4″ (8 to 10 cm); for a child over age 6, advance the tube 2″ to 3″ (5 to 8 cm).

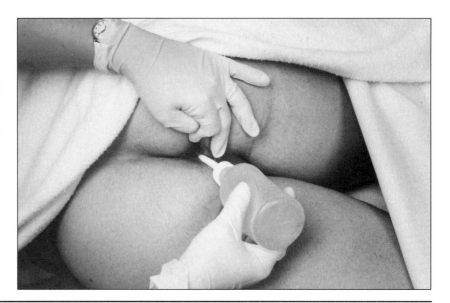

Squeeze the enema container (as shown) until the solution fills the patient's rectum. Remove the rectal tube and discard the used enema and original packaging properly. Tell the patient to retain the solution for the prescribed time.

▷ *Clinical tip:* If the patient is apprehensive, position him on a bedpan, and let him hold toilet tissue or a rolled washcloth against his anus. Place the call button within reach. If he needs to use the bathroom or commode later, instruct him to call for help before getting out of bed, especially if he feels weak or faint.

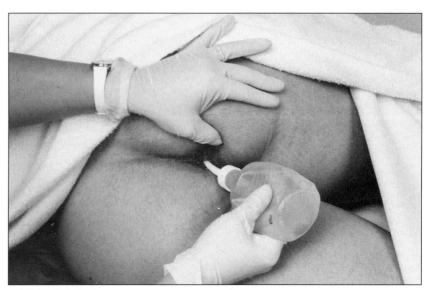

Using an enema bag

Prepare the prescribed enema solution and warm it to 105° F (40.6° C). Test the temperature of the solution with a bath thermometer, or pour a small amount of solution over your wrist. Then put on gloves, close the clamp on the enema tubing (as shown), and fill the enema bag with the solution.

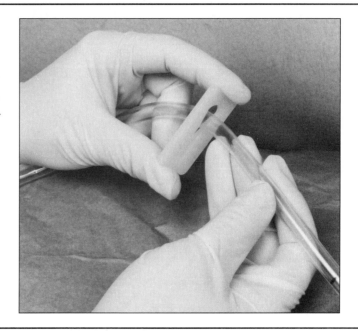

Hang the enema bag on an I.V. pole, adjusting the bag so that it's slightly above bed level.

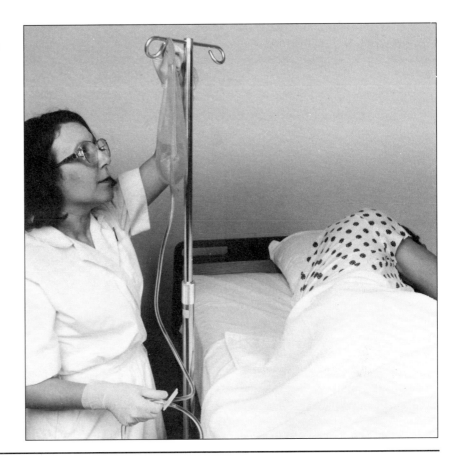

Remove the protective cap from the end of the enema tubing (as shown). The tip of the tubing should be prelubricated. If not, lubricate it with a small amount of water-soluble lubricant.

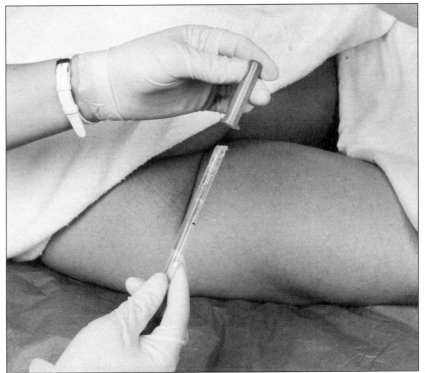

Unclamp the tubing, flush the solution through the tubing, and then reclamp it.

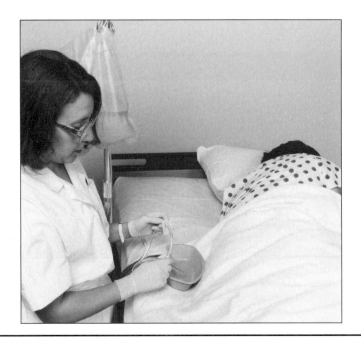

With your nondominant hand, lift the patient's upper buttock. With your other hand, insert the enema tubing into the patient's anus (as shown).

▶ *Clinical tip:* Before inserting the tubing, touch the patient's anal sphincter with the tip of the tube to stimulate contraction. Then, as the sphincter relaxes, tell the patient to breathe deeply through the mouth as you gently advance the tube.

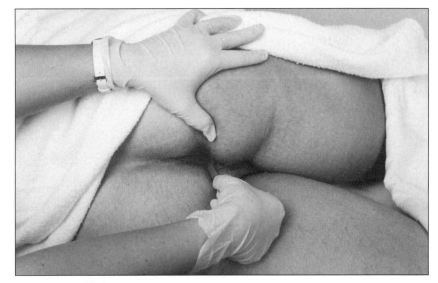

Release the clamp on the tubing. Be sure to hold the tube in place throughout the procedure because bowel contractions and the pressure of the tube against the anal sphincter can lead to tube displacement.

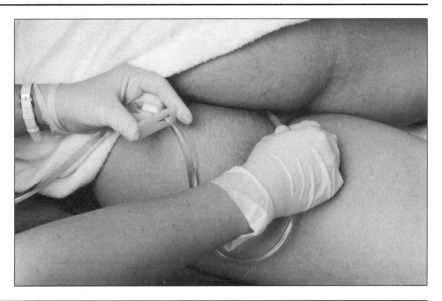

Next, start the flow and adjust the flow rate by lowering or raising the bag according to the patient's retention ability and comfort. However, don't raise it higher than 18″ (46 cm) for an adult, 12″ (30 cm) for a child, and 6″ to 8″ (15 to 20 cm) for an infant.

▶ *Clinical tip:* If the flow stops, the tubing may be blocked with feces or compressed against the rectal wall. Gently turn the tubing slightly to free it without stimulating defecation. If the tubing becomes clogged, withdraw it, flush with solution, and then reinsert.

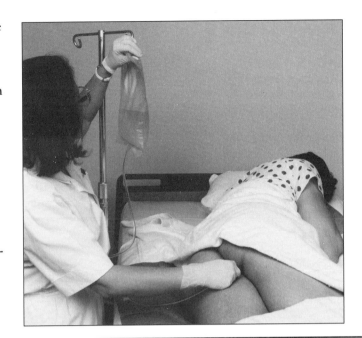

After administering most of the solution, clamp the tubing. Stop the flow before the container empties to avoid introducing air into the bowel. Remove the tubing and dispose of the setup.

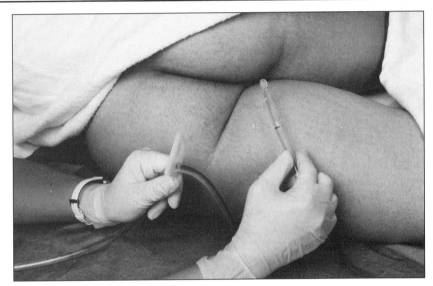

Instruct the patient to hold the solution for the prescribed time. If necessary, hold a 4″ × 4″ gauze pad against the anus until the patient's urge to defecate passes. Place his call button within reach. Place him on a bedpan if doing so will make him more comfortable.

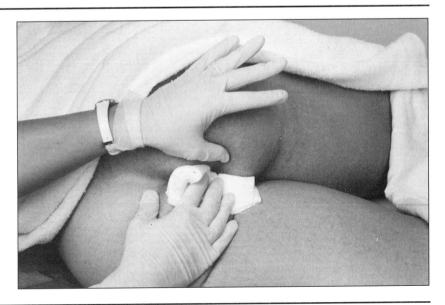

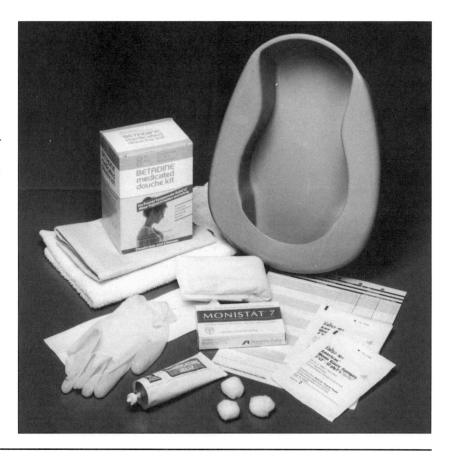

GIVING VAGINAL DRUGS

Among the forms of vaginal drugs are suppositories, creams, gels, ointments, and solutions. These medicated preparations can be inserted to treat infection (particularly *Trichomonas vaginalis* and monilial vaginitis) or inflammation. Or they may be used to prevent conception. Once in contact with the vaginal mucosa, suppositories melt, diffusing medication as effectively as creams, gels, and ointments.

Vaginal medications usually come with a disposable applicator to place the medication in the anterior and posterior fornices. Vaginal administration is most effective when the patient can remain lying down afterward to retain the medication.

Vaginal medications can also be given by irrigation in the form of a douche. The procedure involves instilling a liquid into the vagina at low pressure. The liquid washes the vagina and then immediately flows out without being retained by the patient. Vaginal irrigations can help remove an offensive or irritating discharge, reduce inflammation, or prevent infection.

When performing vaginal irrigation in a hospital, you'll use sterile supplies. In a home setting, sterile technique isn't necessary unless the vagina has an open wound. That's because the vagina isn't a sterile cavity and because patients are usually accustomed to the microorganisms in their homes.

Commercially prepared in prepackaged containers, most vaginal irrigants also come with an insertion nozzle. This nozzle may or may not be already attached to the container.

If a commercially prepared product isn't available, the solution can be instilled through a vaginal irrigation setup. As with other vaginal medications, the best time for administration is bedtime, when the patient can remain lying down.

Vaginal medications may be administered by you or by the patient herself.

Inserting a vaginal drug

Gather the following equipment: the patient's medication record, gloves, water-soluble lubricant, a small sanitary pad, an absorbent towel, a linen-saver pad, a small drape, cotton balls, a 4" × 4" gauze pad, and a paper towel. Soap and water may also be necessary.

To insert medication, you'll also need the prescribed drug and an applicator, if appropriate.

To irrigate the vagina, obtain an irrigation bottle with a nozzle or a vaginal irrigation setup (which includes a nozzle, tubing with a clamp, and a container for the solution) and a bedpan. You'll also need an I.V. pole.

After verifying the medication order, confirm the patient's identity
by asking her name and by checking the name, room number, and
bed number on her wristband.
Wash your hands, explain the procedure to the patient, and provide
privacy. Ask the patient to empty
her bladder.

Help the patient into the lithot-
omy position. Place a linen-saver
pad under her buttocks and a
small drape over her legs. Expose
only her perineum.

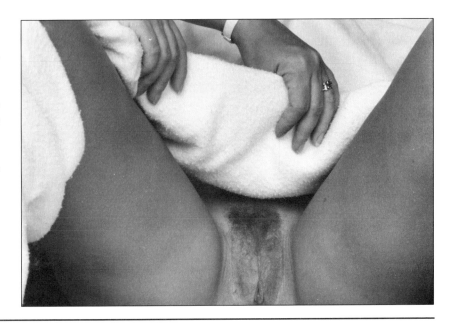

Inserting a vaginal suppository

Wash your hands and put on
gloves. Then squeeze a small portion of water-soluble lubricant on
the 4″ × 4″ gauze pad. Unwrap
the suppository and coat it with
the lubricant.

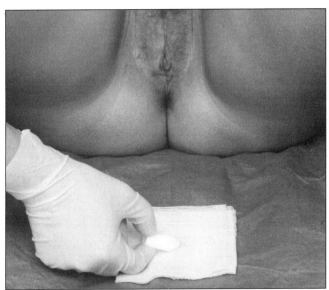

Next, separate the labia. Examine
the patient's perineum. If the perineum is excoriated, withhold the
medication and notify the doctor.
If you see any discharge, wash the
area. To do this, soak several cotton balls in warm, soapy water.
Then, while holding the labia
open with one hand, clean the left
side of the perineum, the right
side and, finally, the center. Use a
fresh cotton ball for each stroke.

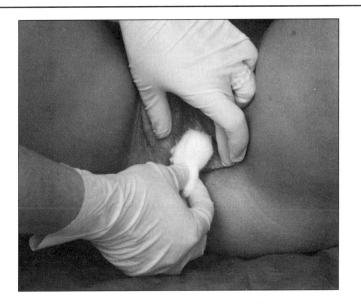

While the patient's labia are still separated, insert the rounded tip of the suppository into her vagina, advancing it about 3″ to 4″ (8 to 10 cm) along the posterior wall of the vagina, or as far as it will go.

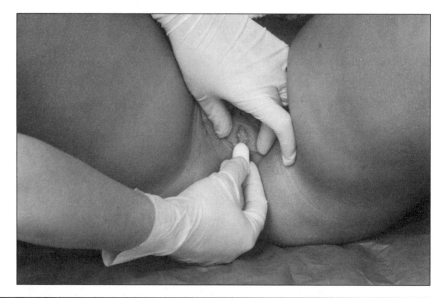

Using an applicator

Medications in the form of a cream, gel, foam, or a small suppository may require the use of an applicator. Some medications come prepackaged in applicators. If not, fill the applicator with the prescribed medication. If the drug is in suppository form, place the suppository in the tip of the applicator. Then, as described above, put on gloves, clean the perineum, and lubricate the applicator tip with water-soluble lubricant.

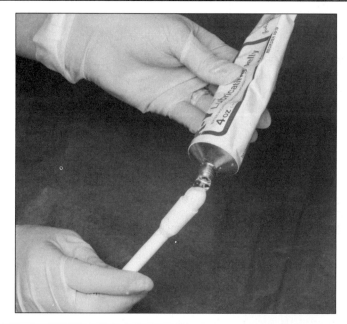

Use your nondominant hand to separate the patient's labia. Use your dominant hand to insert the applicator about 2″ (5 cm) into the patient's vagina.

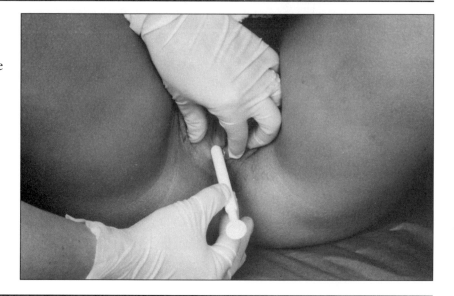

Slowly press the plunger until you empty the applicator.

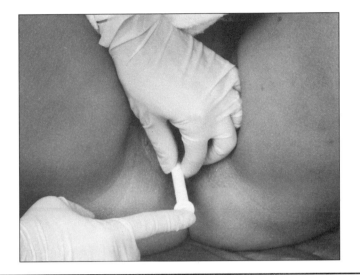

Remove the applicator and place it on a paper towel to prevent the spread of microorganisms. Instruct the patient to remain lying down, with her knees flexed, for 5 to 10 minutes to allow the medication to flow into the posterior fornix. Wash the applicator with soap and warm water and store it or dispose of it as appropriate.

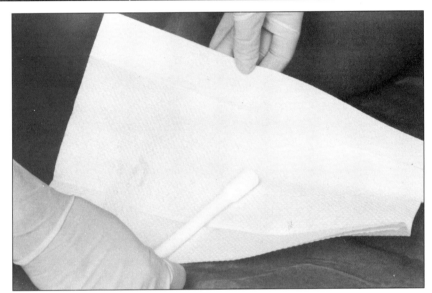

Performing a vaginal irrigation

Prepare the patient as you would to insert a suppository. Then place her on a bedpan, using a pillow or rolled blanket to support her lower back.

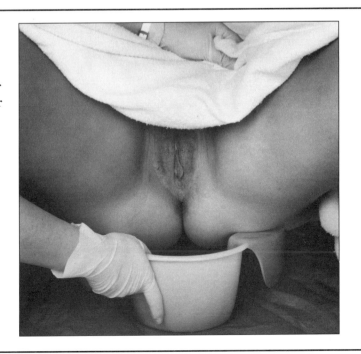

Put on gloves. If necessary, attach the nozzle tip to the irrigation bottle. Remove the protective cap, if applicable, and gently squeeze the bottle to ensure patency of the nozzle tip.

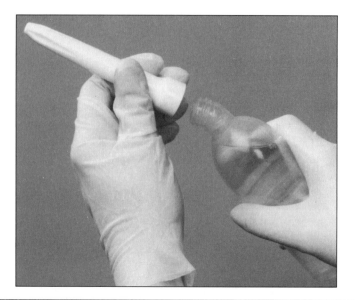

Next, expose the vagina. Insert the nozzle tip as you would an applicator and then squeeze the bottle to instill the solution into the vagina. After infusing into the vagina, the solution should return freely into the bedpan.

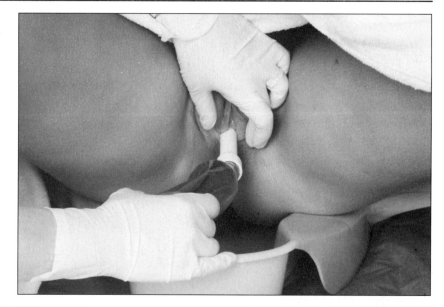

If you'll be assembling an irrigation setup to administer the solution, clamp the irrigation tubing and hang the container of irrigation fluid on the I.V. pole. Adjust the height of the I.V. pole so that the bottom of the solution container is about 12″ (30 cm) above the vagina. This height will allow the solution to flow freely without injuring the vaginal lining.

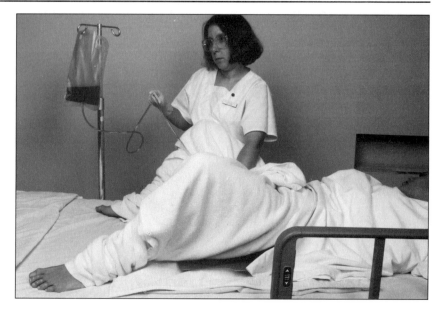

Hold the nozzle over the bedpan and then unclamp the tubing. Allow solution to flow through the tubing to remove air and moisten the nozzle's tip. Then hold the nozzle over the patient's perineum to allow the solution to moisten and clean the perineal area. Clamp the tubing.

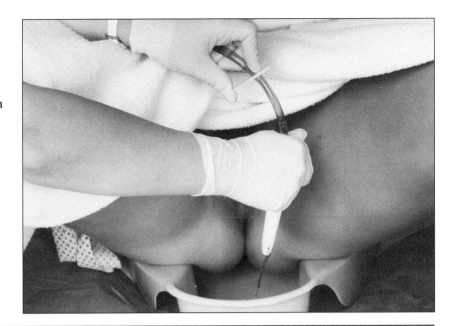

Use your nondominant hand to separate the labia. Use your dominant hand to insert the nozzle into the vagina (as shown). Once the nozzle is inserted, direct it toward the patient's sacrum, and carefully advance it 3″ to 4″ (8 to 10 cm) into the vagina.

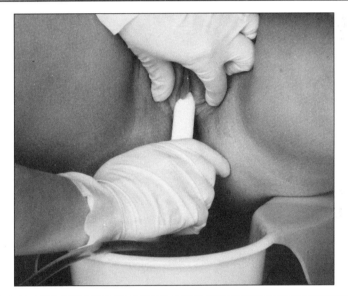

Unclamp the tubing and allow the solution to flow freely into the patient's vagina. Rotate the nozzle several times to irrigate all parts of the vagina.

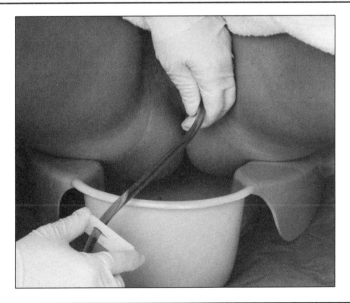

After administering all of the solution, remove the nozzle from the patient's vagina. Remove the bedpan, and pat the patient's perineum and buttocks dry with a towel.

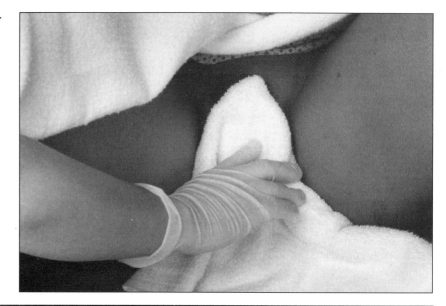

To prevent the medication from soiling the patient's clothing and bedding, provide a sanitary pad. Assist the patient with application, if necessary.

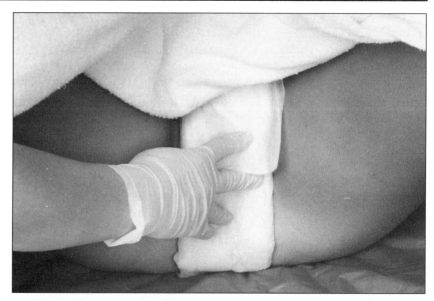

Properly dispose of the irrigation equipment. Then remove your gloves, turning them inside out and placing them on the paper towel. Help the patient return to a comfortable position.

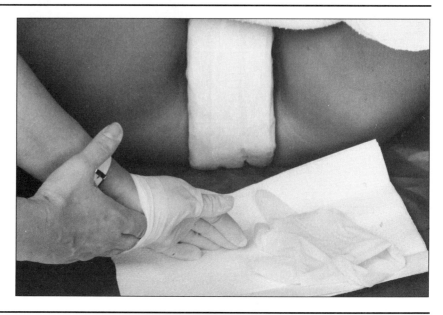

GIVING OPHTHALMIC DRUGS

Ophthalmic drugs—in drop, ointment, disk, or lens form—are diagnostic or therapeutic. An eye patch enhances drug effects and protects ocular tissues.

You'll give eyedrops to anesthetize the eye, dilate the pupil, or stain the cornea (to detect abrasions or scars) during an eye examination. You'll also give eyedrops to lubricate the eye or its socket, protect the vision of a neonate, and treat certain eye disorders—pilocarpine for glaucoma, for example.

The medicated ocular disk stays in the eye and works while the patient sleeps. In contact with the eye's natural fluid, the disk releases medication for up to 1 week. Keep in mind that this device shouldn't be used if the patient has conjunctivitis, keratitis, retinal detachment, or any condition in which pupillary constriction should be avoided.

If your patient has an ocular disk, explain possible adverse effects, such as a foreign-body sensation in the eye, mild tearing or redness, increased mucus discharge, eyelid redness and itching and, possibly, blurred vision, headaches, stinging, and swelling. Reassure her that mild adverse effects are common and should subside within the first 6 weeks of use.

Connected to a 6″ (15-cm) irrigation tube, the Morgan lens is a molded scleral lens that is used to flush an eye or to deliver medication continuously. Fluids and medications can flow through the tubing at a controlled rate and can be stopped or changed without removing the lens. This device may also be used before eye surgery to flush the conjunctiva or during surgery to irrigate and protect the eye. (See *Intervening with the Morgan lens.*)

TAKING PRECAUTIONS

Administer ophthalmic drugs cautiously as follows:
• If you're opening the drug container for the first time, remember to write the date on the label because an opened container should be used within 2 weeks to avoid contamination.
• To prevent contamination, never use a medication container for more than one patient.
• Keep in mind that certain drugs may cause eye disorders or other serious consequences. For example, anticholinergics, which are commonly used during eye examinations, may precipitate acute glaucoma in a predisposed patient.

Intervening with the Morgan lens

CONDITION	INITIAL INTERVENTIONS	ONGOING INTERVENTIONS
Ocular burn	Provide lactated Ringer's solution with antibiotic and steroidal drug added, as ordered. Deliver 500 ml at a rapid, free-flow rate by I.V. infusion.	Continue flow at 50 ml/hour or 15 drops/minute until symptoms subside (usually in 24 to 72 hours).
Ocular injury from gasoline, detergent, or solvent	Provide lactated Ringer's solution with antibiotic and steroidal agents added, as ordered. Deliver 500 ml at a rapid, free-flow rate by I.V. infusion.	Continue infusion at a slower rate, as indicated.
Foreign body sensation (but no visible foreign body)	As ordered, warm 20 ml of sterile water to body temperature. Flush the eye by injecting the solution slowly and gently by syringe.	Repeat once, if indicated.
Severe ocular infection	Provide lactated Ringer's solution with antibiotic and steroidal drug added, as ordered. Infuse at 50 ml/hour or 15 drops/minute.	Continue treatment for 70 hours; then repeat at 10-hour intervals, as ordered.
Preoperative antisepsis	Gently inject 10 ml of an ocular antiseptic by syringe, as ordered.	Administer antiseptic only once.
Eyelid surgery	Give lactated Ringer's solution at 4 drops/minute.	Continue this treatment throughout the surgery.

Mary Jane McDevitt, RN, BS, an oncology nurse at Mercy Catholic Medical Center, Fitzgerald Division, Darby, Pa., contributed to this section. The publisher thanks the following for their help: *Melvyn A. Wolf, MD,* Springhouse, Pa.; *Doylestown (Pa.) Hospital; MorTan, Inc.,* Missoula, Mont.; and *Village Pharmacy at Springhouse (Pa.).*

Administering drops or ointment

To administer eyedrops or an eye ointment, gather the prescribed medication, the patient's medication record, sterile cotton balls, gloves, warm water or 0.9% sodium chloride solution, sterile gauze pads, and facial tissues. You may also need to obtain an eye dressing.

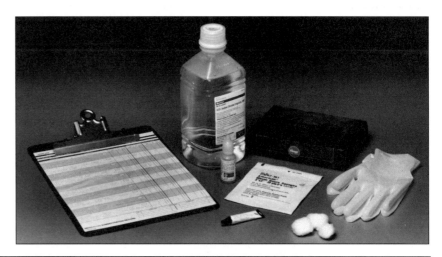

Read the drug label to make sure that the medication is for ophthalmic use. If you're instilling an eyedrop solution, check the expiration date and inspect for cloudiness, discoloration, and precipitates. If the solution appears abnormal in any way, don't use it. If you're administering an ointment and the tip of the tube has crusted, wipe it with a sterile gauze pad to remove the crust. Also be sure to check the expiration date.

▶ *Clinical tip:* Keep in mind that some ophthalmic drugs are in suspension form and normally appear cloudy.

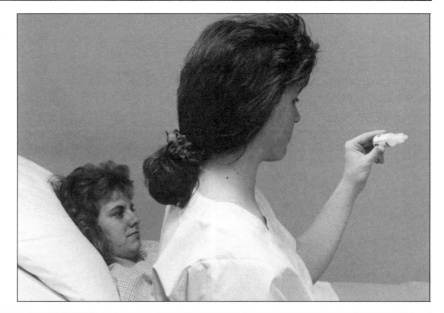

Verify the order on the patient's medication record by checking it against the doctor's order on the patient's chart. Check the medication label against the medication record. Make sure that you know which eye to treat because different medications or dosages may be ordered for each eye. Confirm the patient's identity by asking her name and checking the name, room number, and bed number on her wristband.

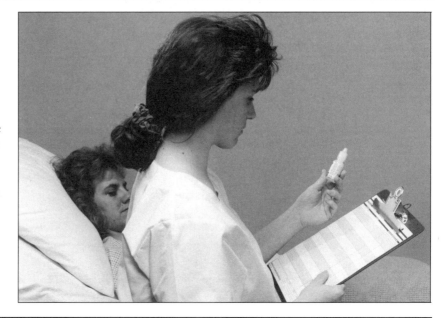

Explain the procedure to the patient and provide privacy. Wash your hands and put on gloves. If the patient has an eye dressing, remove it by gently pulling it down and away from her forehead.

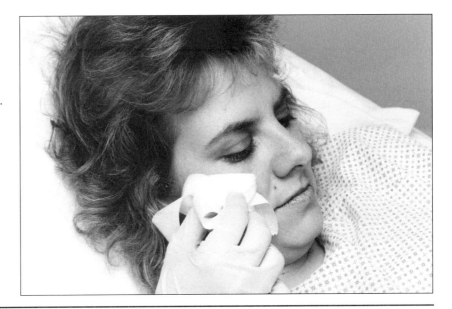

Remove any discharge by cleaning around the eye with sterile cotton balls or sterile gauze pads moistened with warm water or 0.9% sodium chloride solution. Clean from the inner canthus to the outer canthus, using a fresh sterile cotton ball or sterile gauze pad for each stroke.

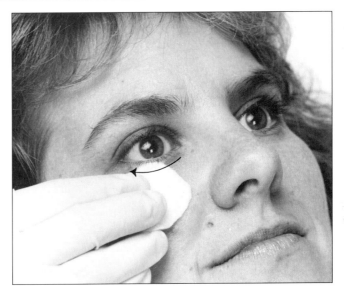

To remove crusted secretions around the eye, moisten a gauze pad with warm water or 0.9% sodium chloride solution. Have the patient close her eye. Then place the moist pad over it for 1 or 2 minutes. Remove the pad and reapply new moist sterile gauze pads, as needed, until the secretions soften enough to be removed without injuring the mucosa.

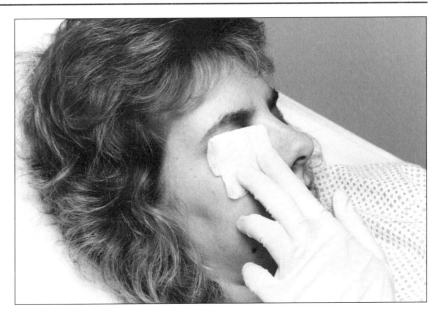

Have the patient tilt her head back and toward the side of the affected eye. This lets excess medication flow away from the tear duct (to minimize systemic absorption). Unless the medication and dropper are a closed unit, remove the dropper cap from the medication bottle and draw the medication into the dropper, taking care not to contaminate it.

▶ *Clinical tip:* Before instilling eyedrops, ask the patient to look up and away. This moves the cornea away from the lower lid and minimizes the risk of touching the cornea with the dropper if the patient blinks.

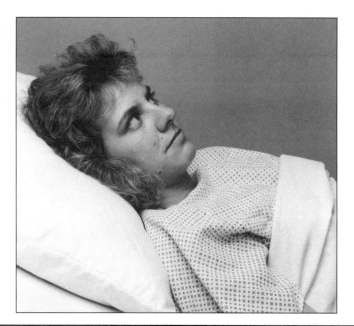

If you're instilling *eyedrops,* steady the hand holding the medication bottle against the patient's forehead. Use your other hand to gently pull down the lower eyelid and instill the drops in the conjunctival sac (as shown), not directly on the eyeball. Release the patient's eyelid, and have her blink to distribute the medication.

▶ *Clinical tip:* Because elderly patients have difficulty sensing drops in the eye, suggest chilling the medication if they'll be instilling it at home. The cold drops should enhance placement sensation.

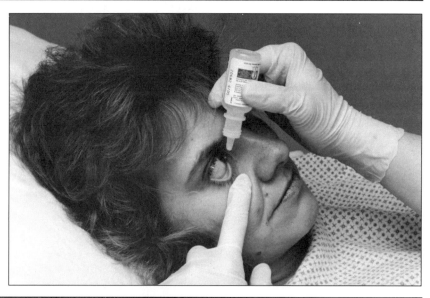

If you're instilling an *eye ointment,* squeeze a small ribbon of medication on the edge of the conjunctival sac from the inner to the outer canthus (as shown). Avoid touching the tube to the patient's eye. Cut off the ribbon by turning the tube. Then release the eyelid and have the patient roll her eyes behind closed lids to distribute the medication.

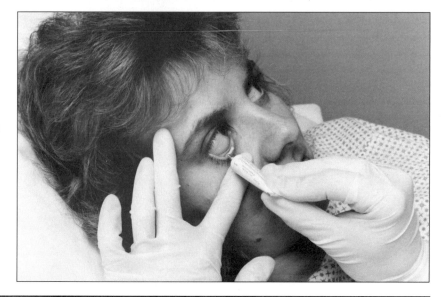

Use a clean tissue to remove any excess solution or ointment leaking from the eye. Use a fresh tissue for each eye to prevent cross-contamination. Finally, apply a new eye dressing if indicated.

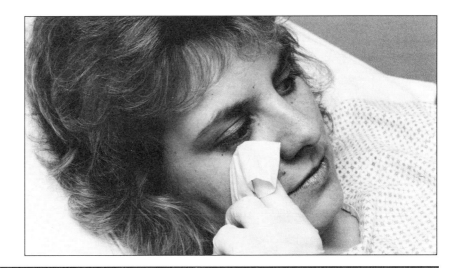

Applying an eye patch

Sometimes after giving an ophthalmic drug, you may need to apply a patch to protect the eye after injury or surgery, to prevent damage to an anesthetized eye, to promote healing, to absorb secretions, or to prevent the patient from touching or rubbing the eye. Or you may need to apply a pressure patch, which is thicker than a conventional patch and requires a doctor's order and supervision. You'll use a pressure patch to promote healing of corneal abrasions, to compress edema, or to control hemorrhage.

Begin by gathering several sterile eye pads, gloves, and tape. You may also need a protective eye shield.

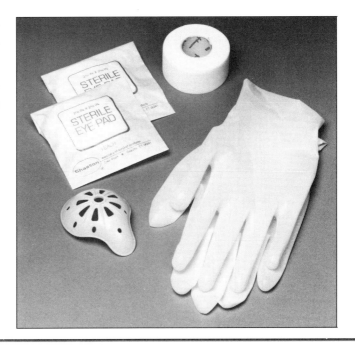

Wash your hands and put on gloves. Explain the procedure to the patient and ask her to close both eyes. Then cover the orbita with a sterile eye pad. Do this by grasping the pad in the center and placing it over the closed eye. This keeps the eyelid from opening.

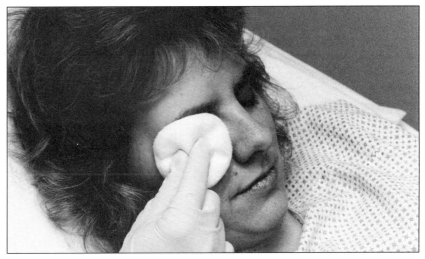

Working from the forehead to the cheekbone, secure the patch with parallel strips of tape (as shown). ▷ *Clinical tip:* If you need to exert pressure or hold the patch in place without tape (in burn injuries, for example), apply a head dressing to secure the patch.

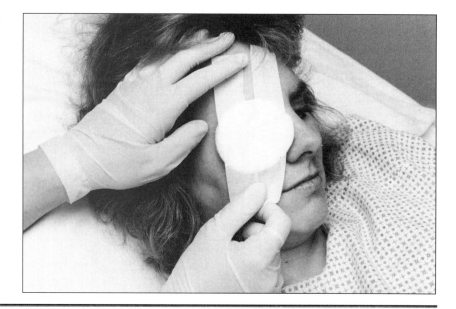

For increased protection of an injured eye, place a plastic shield on top of the eye pad and apply tape over the shield.

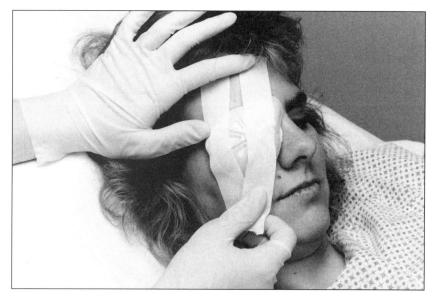

Inserting a medicated disk

Small, flexible, and oval, the medicated ocular disk consists of three layers: two soft outer layers and a middle layer of medication. Inserted in the eye, the disk floats between the eyelid and the sclera. To insert it, you'll need the disk, a cotton-tipped applicator, and gloves.

The best time to insert the disk is just before the patient goes to bed. This eliminates the blurring that usually occurs immediately after disk insertion.

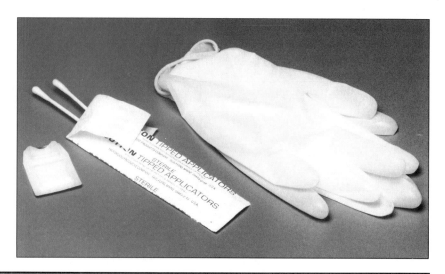

After explaining the procedure to the patient, wash your hands and put on gloves. Place the disk packet in the palm of your non-dominant hand, and press a fingertip of your dominant hand against the oval disk. The disk should stick to your finger length-wise (as shown) as you lift it from its packet.

▶ *Clinical tip:* Rinse your gloved hands well before handling the medication disk. Rinsing will wash away any powder on the gloves, which could irritate the patient's eye. If available, use unpowdered gloves to insert the disk.

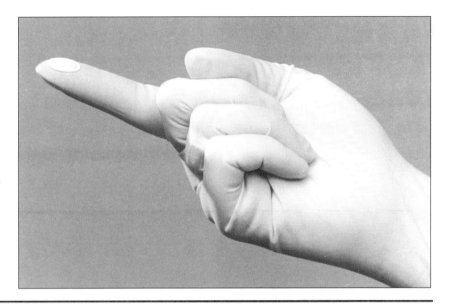

With the finger of your other hand, gently pull the patient's lower eyelid away from her eye. Place the disk in the conjunctival sac (as shown). The disk, which will adhere to the eye naturally, should lie horizontally, not vertically.

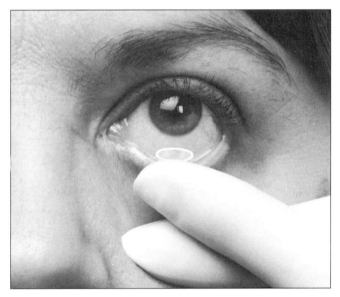

Pull the lower eyelid out, up, and over the disk. Tell the patient to blink several times. If the disk is still visible, pull the lower lid out, up, and over the disk again. If both eyes are being treated with medicated disks, replace both disks at the same time so that both eyes receive medication at the same rate.

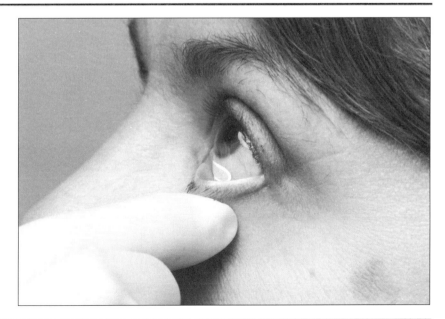

Tell the patient that once the disk is in place, she can adjust its position by gently pressing her finger against her closed eyelid. Caution her against rubbing her eye or moving the disk across the cornea.

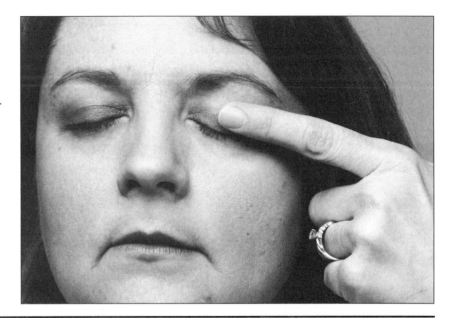

If the disk falls out, wash your hands, put on gloves, rinse the disk in cool water, and reinsert it. If the disk appears bent, however, replace it. If it repeatedly slips out of position, reinsert it in the upper eyelid. To do this, use a cotton-tipped applicator to gently lift and evert the upper eyelid (as shown).

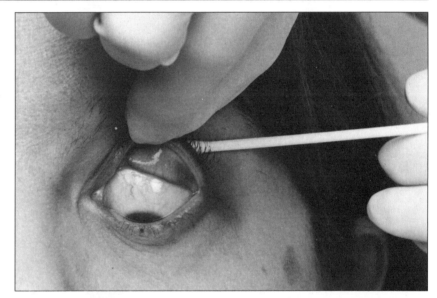

Then insert the medicated disk in the conjunctival sac. Gently pull the eyelid back into position and tell the patient to blink several times. Again, the patient may press gently on the closed eyelid to reposition the disk. The more the patient uses the disk, the easier it should be for her to retain it. If she can't retain it, notify the doctor.

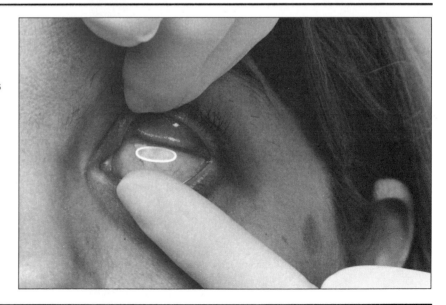

Removing a medicated disk

To remove a disk, put on gloves. In this technique, you use one or two fingers to evert the lower eyelid and expose the disk. Use the forefinger of your other hand to slide the disk onto the lower lid and out of the patient's eye (as shown).

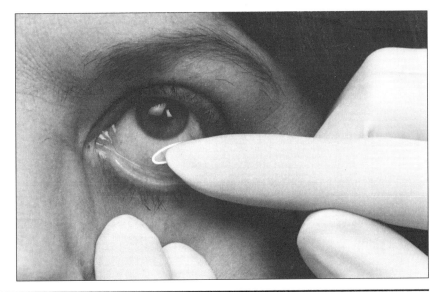

The following removal technique may be easier for you. First, put on gloves. Using two fingers of one hand, evert the lower eyelid to expose the disk. Then pinch the disk with the thumb and forefinger of your other hand and lift it from the eye.

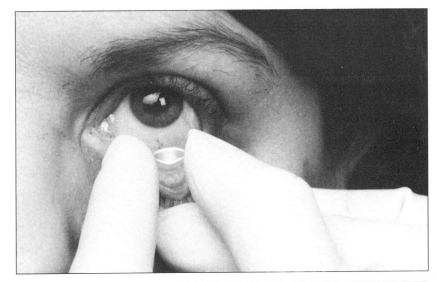

To remove a disk located in the upper eyelid area, apply long, circular strokes to the patient's closed eye with your finger until you see the disk in the corner of the patient's eye. After the disk appears, place your finger directly on it and move it to the lower sclera. Then remove it as you would a disk located in the lower lid area.

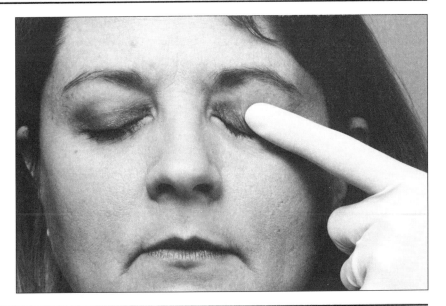

Using the Morgan lens

A patient who has a serious eye injury or infection may need immediate ocular lavage and medication to prevent complications or permanent eye damage. To accomplish this with a Morgan lens, gather these supplies: the lens, sterile gloves, ordered medication or irrigation solution, irrigation tubing (for example, I.V. infusion set tubing), tape, and a topical anesthetic. You may also need tissues or a towel to blot tears and excess solution.

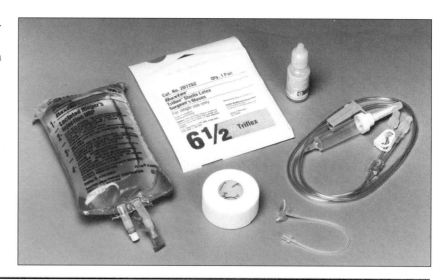

Explain the procedure to the patient, wash your hands, and put on the gloves. As ordered, instill a topical anesthetic into the eye that will receive the Morgan lens.

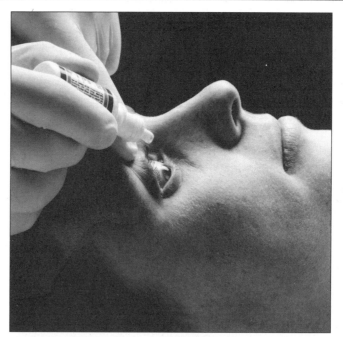

To provide continuous lavage, attach the tubing's adapter to the lens's delivery set or to an I.V. infusion set holding the ordered solution. Then begin the flow to clear the tubing of air.

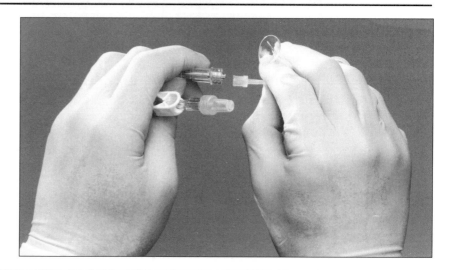

Next, direct the patient to look down. Insert the edge of the lens under the upper lid. Then tell the patient to look up while you retract the lower lid.

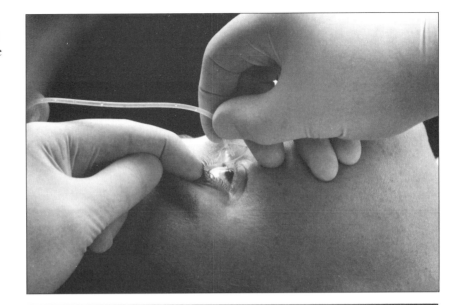

Release the lower lid over the lens to secure the lens in place (as shown). To prevent slippage or accidental lens displacement, you may tape the tubing to the patient's forehead. Wipe off any excess solution with a tissue or a towel.

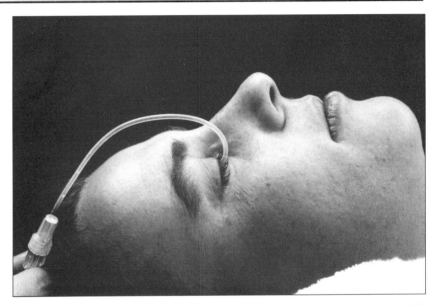

To remove a Morgan lens, ask the patient to look up as you retract the lower lid from the lens's lower border (as shown). While the lower lid is retracted, have the patient look down. Then retract the upper eyelid and slide the lens out.

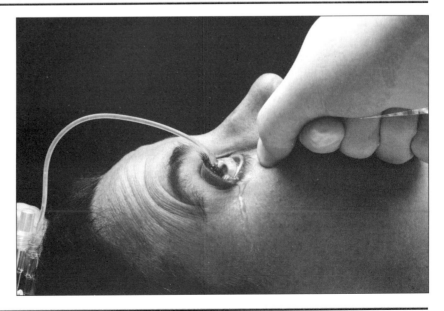

GIVING OTIC DRUGS

Otic drugs may be instilled to treat infections and inflammation, to soften cerumen for later removal, to produce local anesthesia, or to facilitate removal of a foreign object trapped in the ear.

You probably wouldn't instill otic drugs in a patient with a perforated eardrum (although it may be permitted with certain medications and with sterile technique). Certain ear medications may also be prohibited in other conditions because they may enhance the infectious organism's growth—for instance, medications containing hydrocortisone in patients with herpes, another viral infection, or a fungal infection.

Some conditions make the normally sensitive ear canal quite tender, so be especially gentle when instilling ear drugs. Also take special care not to injure the eardrum. Never insert an object, such as a cotton-tipped applicator, into the ear canal past the point where you can see the tip. If the patient has vertigo, keep the side rails of her bed up and assist her as necessary. Also, move slowly to avoid aggravating her vertigo.

Gather the necessary equipment, including the prescribed eardrops, the patient's medication record, a penlight, facial tissues (or cotton-tipped applicators), cotton balls, and an emesis basin for warm water.

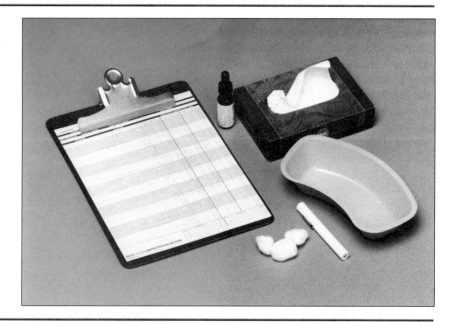

Verify the order on the patient's medication record by checking it against the doctor's order. Then check the medication label against the patient's medication record.

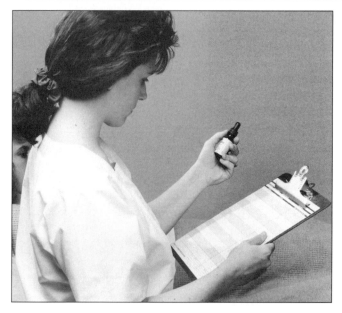

To avoid adverse effects (such as vertigo, nausea, and pain) from instilling eardrops that are too cold, warm the medication to body temperature in the basin of warm water. To avoid burning the patient's eardrum, don't overwarm the medication. If necessary, test the temperature of the medication by placing a drop on your wrist.

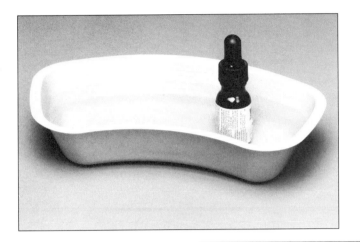

To instill the eardrops, first wash your hands. Confirm the patient's identity by asking her name and checking the name, room number, and bed number on her wristband. Explain the procedure to the patient and provide privacy. Then have the patient lie on her side so that her affected ear faces upward.

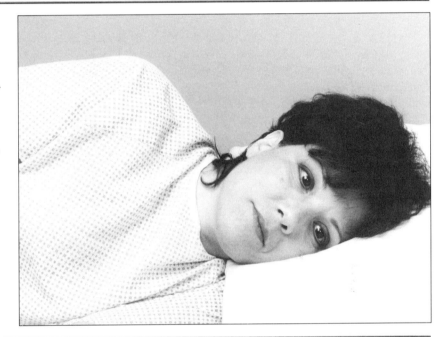

Straighten the patient's ear canal. For an adult, pull the auricle of the ear up and back (near right).

▶ *Clinical tip:* For an infant or a child under age 3, gently pull the auricle down and back (far right) because the ear canal is positioned differently in infants and toddlers.

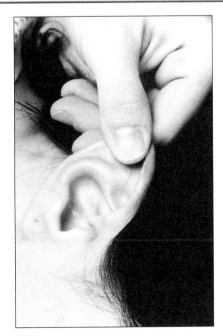
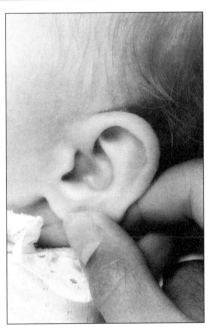

Using the penlight, examine the ear canal for drainage (as shown). If you find any, clean the canal with a tissue or cotton-tipped applicator because drainage can reduce the medication's effectiveness.

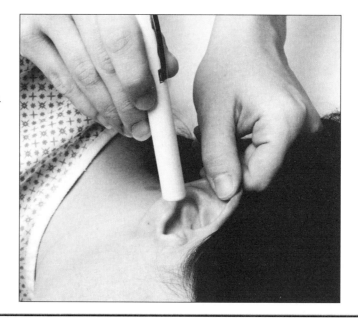

Straighten the patient's ear canal once again and instill the ordered number of drops. To avoid patient discomfort, aim the dropper so that the drops fall against the sides of the ear canal, not on the eardrum. Hold the ear canal in position until you see the medication disappear down the canal. Then release the ear.

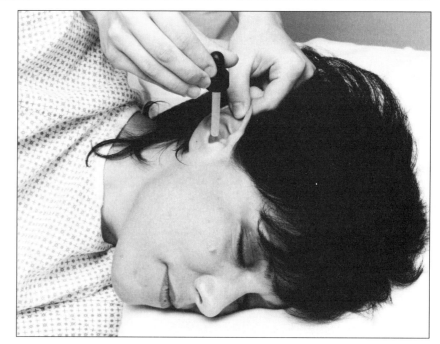

Instruct the patient to remain on her side for 5 to 10 minutes to allow the medication to travel down the ear canal. If ordered, tuck a cotton ball loosely into the opening of the ear canal to contain the medication. Avoid inserting it too deeply because this would prevent secretions from draining and increase pressure on the eardrum.

  Then clean and dry the outer ear. Assist the patient into a comfortable position and wash your hands.

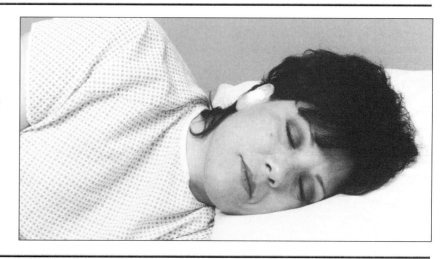

Giving Injections and Infusions

GIVING AN INTRADERMAL INJECTION

An intradermal injection delivers small amounts of a drug or an antigen (usually 0.5 ml or less) into the outer, superficial layers of the skin. Commonly performed to determine antigenic sensitivity by stimulating an immune response, an intradermal injection is used to produce a local effect, known as a wheal. Little systemic absorption occurs.

Intradermal injection allows identification of antibodies to such pathogens as the tubercle bacillus. For some patients, the doctor may order a local anesthetic injected intradermally before venipuncture, although the practice isn't endorsed by the Intravenous Nurses Society.

If you're using an intradermal injection of lidocaine as the anesthetic, you'll administer only a small amount, and it will work in 2 to 3 seconds. Lidocaine injected intradermally numbs pain but allows the patient to feel touch and pressure.

REVIEWING COMMON INJECTION SITES

The most common site for an intradermal injection is the ventral forearm because it's easily accessed and relatively hairless. For extensive allergy testing, the shoulder blades and the outer aspect of the upper arms may also be used.

Gather the necessary equipment: a tuberculin syringe with a 26G or 27G ½" or ⅝" needle, the prescribed test antigen (or drug), gloves, a marking pen, alcohol sponges, and the patient's medication record. Verify the order on the patient's medication record by comparing it to the doctor's order.

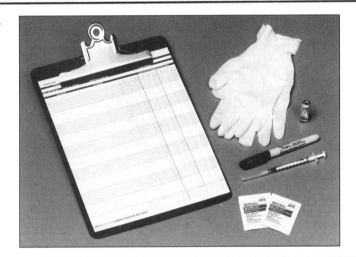

Prepare the medication, comparing the label with the medication record to be sure that you're giving the right drug. Verify the patient's identity by checking the name, room number, and bed number on her wristband.

Tell the patient where you'll give the injection. If it will be in the ventral forearm (shown), instruct her to sit up. Then ask her to extend her arm and support it with the ventral surface exposed.

Mention that she'll need to stay nearby for about 30 minutes after the injection (in case of anaphylaxis).

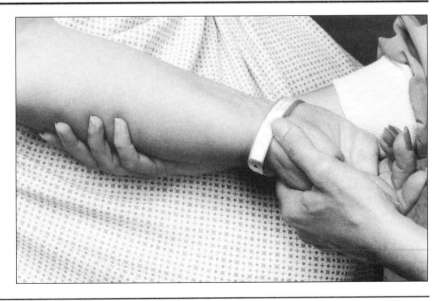

Contributors to this section include *Mary Jane McDevitt, RN, BS,* an oncology staff nurse at Mercy Catholic Medical Center, Fitzgerald Mercy Division, Darby, Pa., and *Claire Keane, RN, MSN,* an assistant professor at Bucks County Community College, Newtown, Pa. The publisher thanks *Doylestown (Pa.) Hospital* and *Delcrest Medical Products,* Blue Bell, Pa., for their help.

Put on gloves. With an alcohol sponge, clean the surface of the ventral forearm about two or three fingerbreadths distal to the antecubital space. Make sure that the test site is free of hair and blemishes. Allow the skin to dry completely before giving the injection.

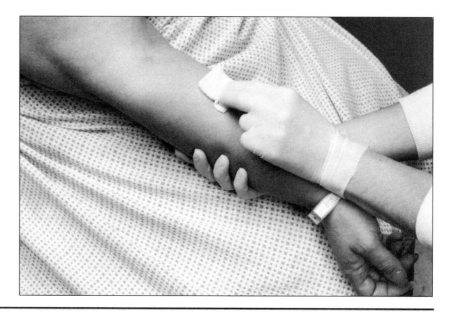

Holding the patient's forearm in your nondominant hand, stretch the skin taut.

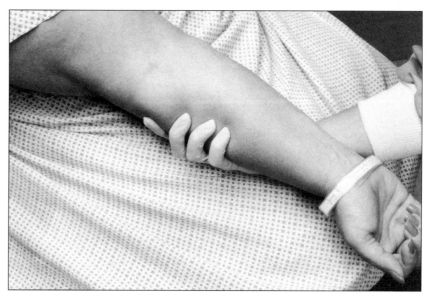

With your dominant hand, hold the needle at a 15-degree angle to the patient's arm, with the bevel facing up.

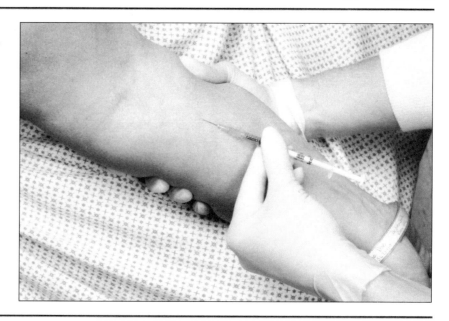

Insert the needle about ⅛" (3 mm) below the epidermis. Stop when the needle's bevel tip is under the skin. Then gently inject the antigen. You should feel some resistance as you do this, and a wheal should form. If no wheal forms, you've probably injected the antigen too deeply. Withdraw the needle and administer another test dose at least 2" (5 cm) from the first site. If you're giving additional injections, be sure to space them about 2" apart.

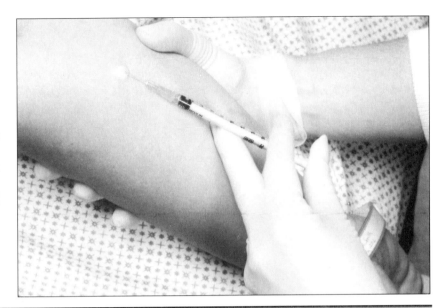

Withdraw the needle at the same angle at which you inserted it. Do not rub the site. This could irritate the underlying tissue, which could affect test results.

▶ *Clinical tip:* A patient who's hypersensitive to the test antigen may have a severe anaphylactic reaction. Be prepared to inject epinephrine immediately and to perform other emergency resuscitation procedures.

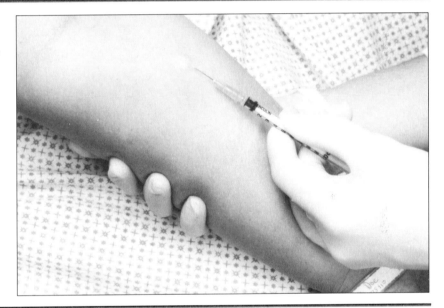

Circle each test site with a marking pen, and label each site to recall the antigen given. Instruct the patient to refrain from washing off the markings until the test period ends. Dispose of needles and syringes according to hospital policy. Remove and discard your gloves. Finally, document the name of the medication or antigen and the amount administered.

Have the patient stay nearby for 30 minutes after testing to allow you to observe for anaphylaxis. Notify the doctor immediately if an allergic reaction occurs. In most cases, a reaction occurs within 72 hours.

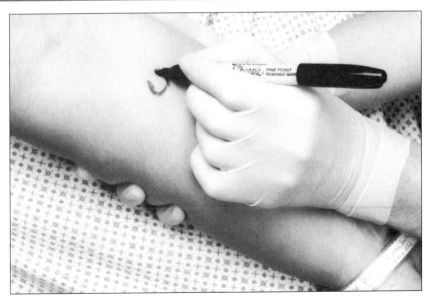

INSIGHTS AND INTERPRETATIONS

Reading skin test results

Follow these general guidelines for reading skin test results easily and confidently:
• Feel the area around the injection site. It should be round and hard (indurated). At the same time, observe the skin for flare (erythema), assessing its extent if present. Keep in mind that erythema without induration isn't significant.
• Measure the extent of the induration in millimeters.
• Record your findings.

Specific guidelines for reading tuberculin and allergy test results follow.

Reading tuberculin test results

When testing for tuberculosis (TB), use a scale (such as the one shown below) to measure the findings.
• If the induration is smaller than 5 mm in diameter, consider the test result negative.
• If the induration is 5 mm or more in diameter, consider the test result positive in any of the following circumstances:
— The patient had recent close contact with a person with active, infectious TB.
— The patient's chest X-ray shows pulmonary fibrotic lesions suggesting old healed TB lesions.
— The patient has human immunodeficiency virus (HIV) or is at high risk for it.
• If the induration is 10 mm or more in diameter, consider the test result positive if the patient fails to meet the above criteria but meets one or more of the following risk factors for TB:
— a medical condition that increases the patient's risk for active TB after infection has occurred (for example, chronic obstructive pulmonary disease or acquired immunodeficiency syndrome)
— birthplace in Asia, Africa, Central America, or South America
— Black, Native American, or Hispanic *and* a member of a low socioeconomic or medically underserved group
— I.V. drug use
— resident or staff member of a congregate living arrangement, such as a prison, nursing home, or other long-term care facility
— health care worker exposed to TB
— extreme youth or old age.
• If the induration is 15 mm or more in diameter, consider the test result positive even if the patient has no risk factors.

Note: A positive skin test result indicates that the patient has been infected with *Mycobacterium tuberculosis.* It does not necessarily indicate active disease.

Reading allergy test results

When testing for allergies, score the findings from 0 to 4+, as follows:
• If the induration is 2 mm or less in diameter, score the test result as 0 (negative).
• If the induration (with erythema) is 3 to 5 mm in diameter, the test score will be 1+.
• If the induration (with erythema) is 6 to 10 mm in diameter, the test score will be 2+.
• If the induration (with erythema) is round and 11 to 15 mm (or more) in diameter, the test score will be 3+.
• If the induration (with erythema) exceeds 15 mm in diameter and has pseudopods (asymmetrical branches), the test score will be 4+.

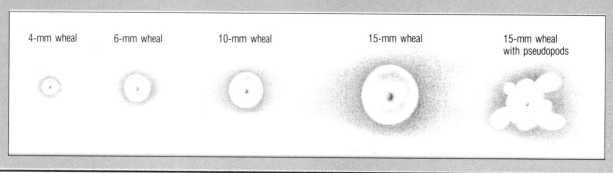

GIVING A SUBCUTANEOUS INJECTION

A drug injected subcutaneously (S.C.) into the adipose (fatty) tissue beneath the skin reaches the bloodstream more quickly than a drug taken by mouth. S.C. injection also allows slower, more sustained drug absorption than intramuscular injection. What's more, this method causes minimal tissue trauma and poses little risk of injuring large blood vessels and nerves.

Absorbed mainly through the capillaries, drugs recommended for S.C. injection include nonirritating aqueous solutions and suspensions contained in 0.5 to 2 ml of fluid. Give drugs and solutions for S.C. injection through a short needle, using sterile technique. You can give S.C. injections in any part of the body that has relatively few sensory nerve endings and no bones or large blood vessels near the surface. (See *Locating S.C. injection sites.*)

Although heparin and insulin are usually administered S.C., you'll need to modify your procedure slightly when giving these drugs. Because these drugs are commonly given at least once daily, you'll need to rotate injection sites. To ensure consistent blood levels, use specific sites because the absorption rate varies from one anatomic region to another. When giving heparin S.C., for instance, the designated administration site is the lower abdominal fat pad just below the umbilicus.

Avoid giving S.C. injections at sites that are inflamed, edematous, scarred, or covered by a mole, a birthmark, or another lesion. Such injections may also be contraindicated in patients with coagulation defects.

Locating S.C. injection sites

Indicated by dotted areas in the photographs, S.C. injection sites include the fat pads on the abdomen, upper hips, upper back, and lateral upper arms and thighs.

For drugs that must be administered repeatedly, such as insulin, rotate the sites. Choose one injection site in one area, move to a corresponding injection site in the next area, and so on. When returning to an area, choose a new site in that area. Preferred injection sites for insulin are the arms, abdomen, thighs, and upper hips.

Heparin administration sites differ from other S.C. injection sites because this drug should be injected only in the lower abdominal fat pad, about 2″ (5 cm) beneath the iliac crests. Administration at this site reduces local capillary bleeding.

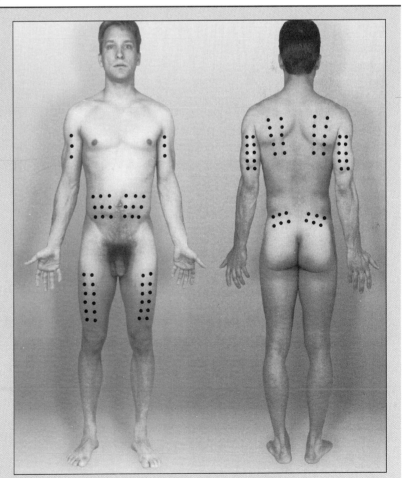

Assemble the equipment you'll need: the prescribed medication, the patient's medication record, a needle of appropriate gauge and length (usually a 25G ⅝″ needle for an average adult and a 25G to 27G ½″ needle for an infant, a child, or an elderly or thin patient), gloves, a 1- to 3-ml syringe, and alcohol sponges. Optional supplies include an antiseptic cleaning agent, a filter needle, and an insulin syringe.

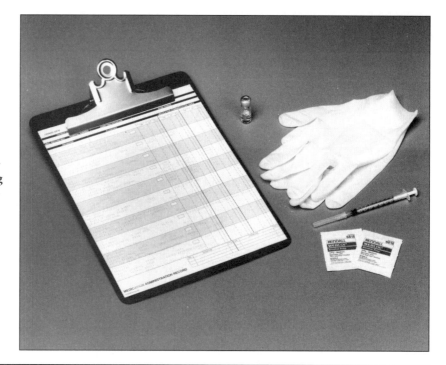

Obtain the prescribed medication, and check it against the medication record and the doctor's order. Prepare the medication, comparing the label with the medication record to be sure that you're giving the right drug. Verify the patient's identity by checking his wristband. Then inspect the medication (as shown) to make sure that it's not abnormally discolored or cloudy and that it doesn't contain precipitates.

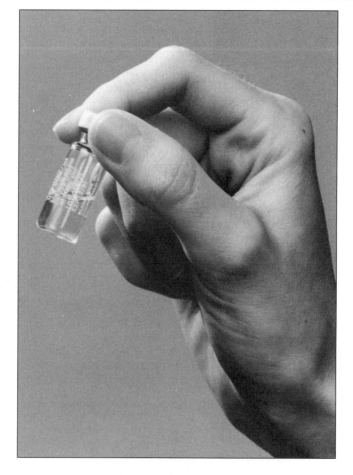

Select an appropriate injection site, remembering to rotate the site if the patient's schedule requires repeated injections. Use different body areas unless contraindicated by the drug. Also select a needle of proper gauge and length. To determine the needle size exactly, use your thumb and forefinger to form a fold of skin at the site (as shown). Measure the fold from base to crest. If it measures more or less than ⅝" (1.6 cm), remove the ⅝" needle from the syringe and replace it with one that's closer to the correct length.

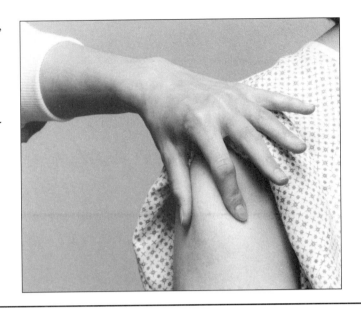

Put on gloves. Position and drape the patient if necessary. Clean the injection site with an alcohol sponge, beginning at the center of the site and moving outward in a circular motion (as shown). Allow the skin to dry before injecting the drug to avoid a stinging sensation from introducing alcohol into S.C. tissue.

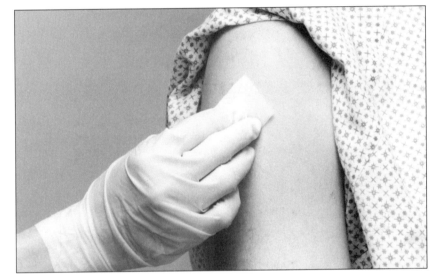

Grasp the skin firmly. This elevates the S.C. tissue and prevents the needle from entering the wrong skin layer.

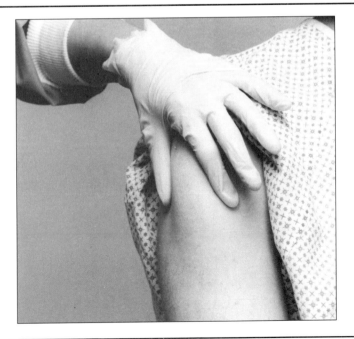

Position the needle with the bevel facing up. If you're using a ⅝″ or longer needle, hold it at a 45-degree angle (near right). If you're injecting the drug with a ½″ needle, hold it at a 90-degree angle (far right). Insert the needle with one quick motion; then release your grasp on the patient's skin. If you don't, you'll inject the drug into the compressed tissue, which will irritate nerve fibers and cause discomfort.

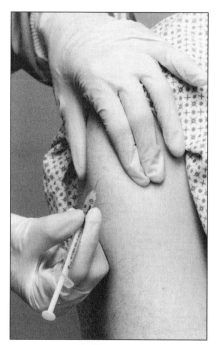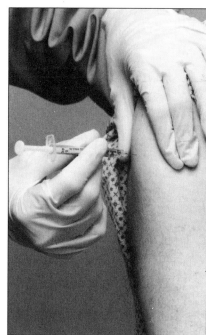

Pull back slightly on the plunger to check needle placement. If no blood flows back into the syringe, begin injecting the drug slowly. If blood appears upon aspiration, withdraw the needle, prepare another syringe, and repeat the procedure.

▶ *Clinical tip:* Don't aspirate for blood return when giving insulin or heparin. Aspiration isn't necessary with insulin and may cause a hematoma with heparin.

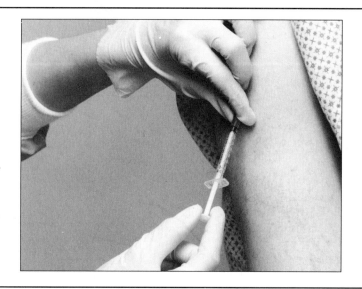

After injection, remove the needle gently but quickly at the same angle used for insertion. Cover the site with an alcohol sponge. Then massage the site gently (unless you have injected a drug that contraindicates massage, such as heparin or insulin) to distribute the drug and facilitate absorption. Dispose of used equipment according to hospital policy. To avoid needle-stick injuries, don't resheath the needle. Finish up by documenting the procedure.

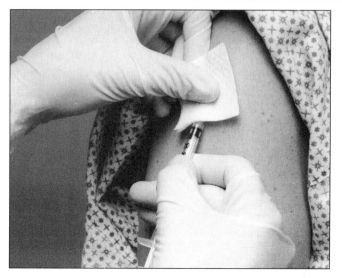

IMPLANTING GOSERELIN CAPSULES IN THE ABDOMEN

A patient with prostate cancer or endometriosis may benefit from a recently developed therapy using goserelin, a synthetic form of luteinizing hormone–releasing hormone (LHRH)—also known as gonadotropin-releasing hormone. Normally, the hypothalamus releases this hormone, which triggers the pituitary gland to release luteinizing hormone (LH) in men and follicle-stimulating hormone (FSH) in women.

In men, LH causes the testes to produce testosterone; an injection of goserelin produces the same effect. At first, testosterone production surges, which may worsen the symptoms of prostate cancer, such as dysuria or urine retention. However, within 2 to 4 weeks, goserelin suppresses testosterone production.

In women, FSH causes the ovaries to release estradiol. An injection of goserelin suppresses serum estradiol levels and, in turn, decreases the formation of endometrial tissue. The result: reduction of such symptoms as pelvic pain, dysmenorrhea, and dyspareunia.

A timesaving way to implant goserelin (Zoladex) in the subcutaneous tissue is currently available. The hormone comes prepared in a 1-cm-long capsule for injection into the anterior abdominal wall through a needle-syringe device. Completely biodegradable, the capsule is slowly absorbed by the body over 28 days. Injections are repeated for as long as the patient has prostate cancer or for 6 months if the patient has endometriosis. Hormone levels gradually return to normal after therapy ends.

Begin by gathering the equipment, including a goserelin implant (shown out of its sterile pouch and package) in its needle-syringe device.

You'll also need an alcohol sponge, an adhesive bandage, gloves, 4″ × 4″ gauze pads, and a biohazard container for the needle and syringe.

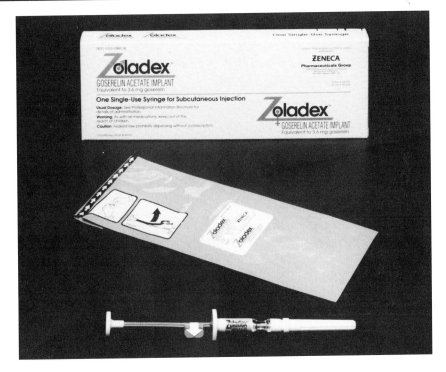

Karen E. Michael, RN, MSN, a case manager with Greater Atlantic Health Service in Philadelphia, contributed to this section. The publisher thanks *Hill-Rom,* Batesville, Ind., and *Zeneca Pharmaceuticals,* Wilmington, Del., for their help.

Verify the order on the patient's medication record by checking it against the doctor's order. Explain the procedure to the patient and place the equipment at his bedside. Then wash your hands.

Examine the goserelin implant's sterile foil package for damage. Then open the package, remove the syringe, and make sure that the implant is visible in the syringe's translucent chamber (as shown). If the pouch or syringe appears damaged, obtain a replacement.

Next, confirm the patient's identity by checking his identification band. Then provide privacy and help him into a supine position.

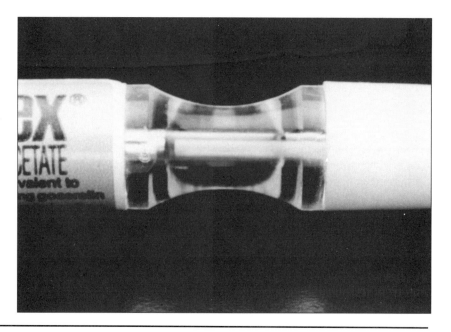

Assess the subcutaneous fat in the patient's abdominal area by gently grasping the tissue between your thumb and index finger. Expect the skin fold to be pliable and soft with at least ½″ (1.3 cm) of fat. If it doesn't meet these requirements, withhold the injection and consult the doctor.

Select an injection site in one of the abdominal quadrants. The site should be at least 2″ (5 cm) away from the umbilicus and free of rashes, bruises, or scars. Put on gloves and clean the selected site with an alcohol sponge. Start in the center and, using a circular motion, wipe outward.

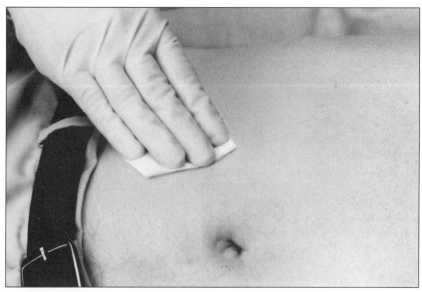

After preparing the injection site, withdraw the syringe from its wrapper, remove the red plastic safety clip on the plunger (as shown), and take off the needle cover.

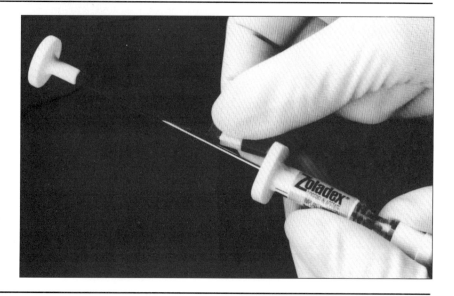

Use your nondominant hand to gently pinch the patient's abdominal tissue, taking care to grasp enough tissue to provide a flat surface with adequate subcutaneous tissue.

Holding the barrel of the syringe in your dominant hand, begin to insert the needle with the bevel facing up at a 45-degree angle. Stop advancing the needle when the bevel rests in subcutaneous tissue.

▶ *Clinical tip:* Do not aspirate. This syringe can't be used for aspiration. If the needle should penetrate a large vessel, blood will instantly leak into the syringe chamber.

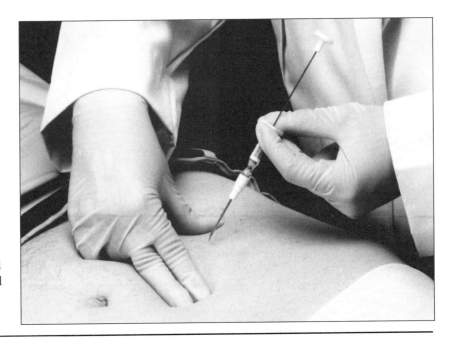

Lower the syringe until the needle is parallel to the abdominal wall, and continue inserting the needle until the barrel's hub touches the patient's skin.

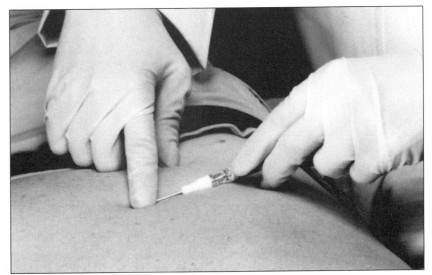

Next, withdraw the needle ½" (1.3 cm) to create a space for the implant; then push the syringe's plunger to inject the implant into that space.

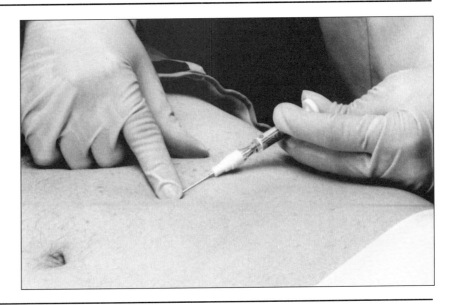

Remove the needle and, using a 4″ × 4″ gauze pad, apply pressure at the injection site for 30 seconds.

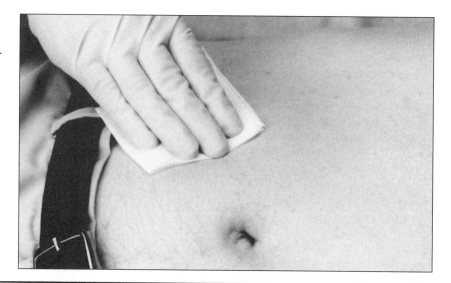

Apply an adhesive bandage over the injection site. Then examine the tip of the needle. If the implant was fully discharged, you should see the end of the plunger at the tip of the needle (as shown).

Discard the needle and syringe in the appropriate container in accordance with your hospital's policy. Remove your gloves, wash your hands, and document the procedure (making sure that you include the name of the medication, the dose, the time and date of implantation, the injection site, and the patient's response).

Also, monitor the injection site for bleeding or bruising, and instruct the patient about possible adverse effects, such as hot flashes, sexual dysfunction, and headaches. Advise him to contact his doctor if these effects are severe.

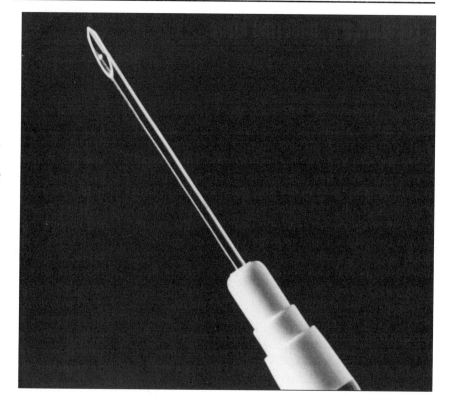

GIVING INSULIN THROUGH AN IMPLANTED CATHETER

Today's technological advances allow patients who require frequent insulin injections to receive them through an indwelling subcutaneous catheter (such as the Insuflon catheter featured below). This kind of catheter can be used in adults and children to administer insulin for 3 to 7 days, sparing the patient repeated needle sticks.

The device, consisting of an 18-mm catheter over a 24G 19-mm needle, is inserted beneath the abdominal skin, and the needle withdrawn. The catheter then remains embedded in the subcutaneous tissue. Although the soft plastic tubing seldom causes irritation, it isn't recommended for people who are prone to skin infections or for those who are allergic to adhesive tape.

An adhesive-backed foam disk with an opening in the center covers the catheter's wings and the insertion site. It also secures the catheter. The opening in the disk is covered with transparent film for easy viewing of the insertion site.

After insertion, the catheter should be removed every 3 to 5 days and a new one inserted on the opposite side of the abdomen about 1″ to 2″ (2.5 to 5 cm) away from other recently used sites on that side. The catheter can remain in place for up to 7 days if the patient's skin stays free of irritation.

Inserting the catheter

To prepare the Insuflon catheter for use, you'll need an Insuflon package (containing the needle-catheter assembly and an adhesive-backed foam disk), gloves, and an alcohol sponge.

To administer insulin after inserting the catheter, you'll need the insulin, an insulin syringe, alcohol sponges, and another pair of gloves.

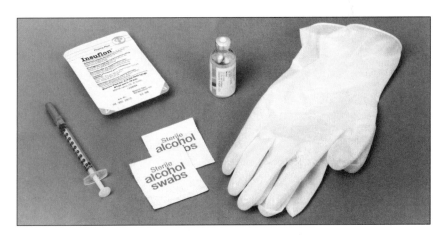

Explain the procedure to the patient, wash your hands, and examine the patient's skin for an insertion site. The abdomen (or the area used for regular insulin injections) is usually the best site. Avoid placing the catheter in skin folds or in areas where clothing may rub against it.

Next, open the sterile Insuflon package. Put on clean gloves, choose the insertion site, and clean it with an alcohol sponge. Using a circular pattern, wipe from the center outward. Allow the area to dry (up to 2 minutes).

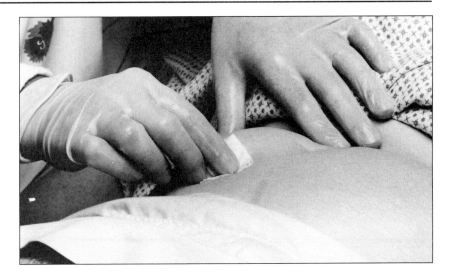

Karen E. Michael, RN, MSN, a case manager with Greater Atlantic Health Service in Philadelphia, contributed to this section. The publisher thanks *Hill-Rom*, Batesville, Ind., and *Chronimed Inc.*, Minnetonka, Minn., for their help.

Hold the catheter assembly by the wings, and remove the protective cap from the needle.

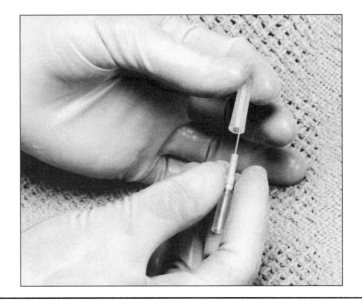

Place the cap in the back of the device, being careful not to touch the sterile needle.

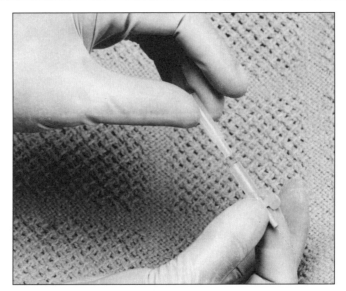

Hold the device behind the wings (as if you're holding a pen), and pinch up the skin at the insertion site.

▶ *Clinical tip:* Don't grip the wings during insertion. This could cause the needle to puncture the catheter.

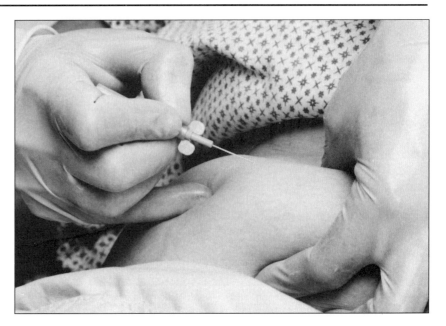

Using just one quick motion, insert the device into the subcutaneous tissue at a 45-degree angle so that the wings lie flat against the skin.

▶ *Clinical tip:* Avoid inserting the device slowly. Doing so may cause the catheter to peel back along the steel needle.

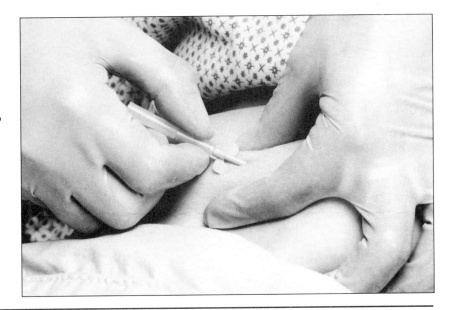

Remove the needle by holding the wings with one hand and pulling the needle out with the other hand. Make sure the catheter stays under the skin.

▶ *Clinical tip:* Never try to reinsert a partially or completely withdrawn needle. The needle could tear the catheter.

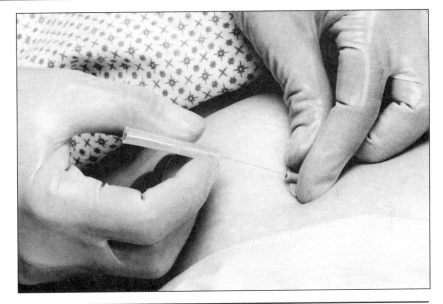

Peel the adhesive-backed foam disk from the backing, and leave it sticky-side up on the table.

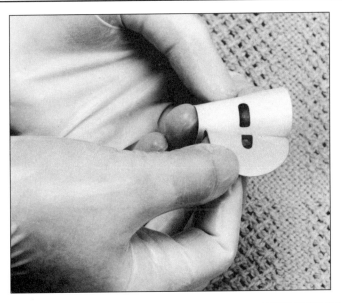

Cover the catheter from the insertion site to the injection port with the adhesive-backed foam disk. Apply the arrowhead end of the adhesive over the insertion site first, making sure that the site is clearly visible through the arrowhead's transparent opening (as shown). Then apply the open rectangular end over the distal end of the catheter.

Next, remove your gloves and wash your hands. Document the procedure in the medical record. Identify the insertion site and describe the patient's response.

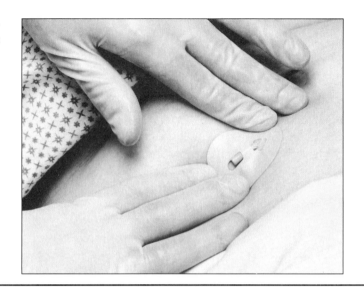

Delivering the insulin

Verify the insulin order in the patient's chart. Also check the result of his last blood glucose test (if applicable). Explain the procedure to the patient, wash your hands, and put on gloves. Wipe the film over the catheter port with an alcohol sponge and allow the alcohol to dry.

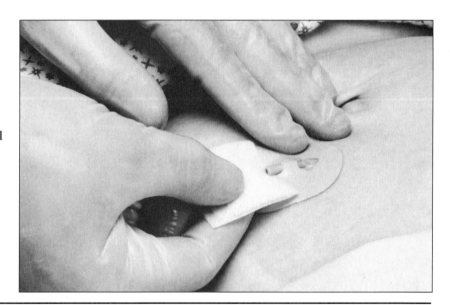

Insert the needle of the insulin syringe into the center of the catheter's port membrane. Insert it at least ¼", but no more than ⅜", because doing so could puncture the catheter.

▶ *Clinical tip:* If you're having difficulty inserting the needle, try rotating it as you insert it into the port.

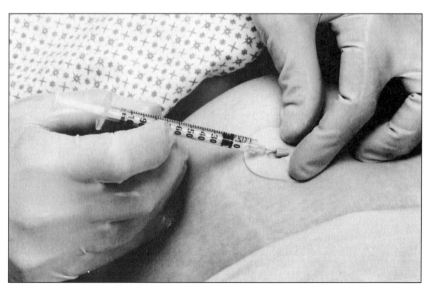

Depress the plunger to inject the insulin into the catheter, and remove the needle. Dispose of the needle in the appropriate container. Document the medication, the dose, the date and time of insertion, and the insertion site in the medication record.

▶ *Clinical tip:* Studies show that about 0.5 unit of the first insulin injection is lost to the patient because it remains in the catheter. The loss is usually negligible. To make up for it, however, you may want to obtain a doctor's order to add an extra unit of insulin to the first dose delivered after each catheter insertion.

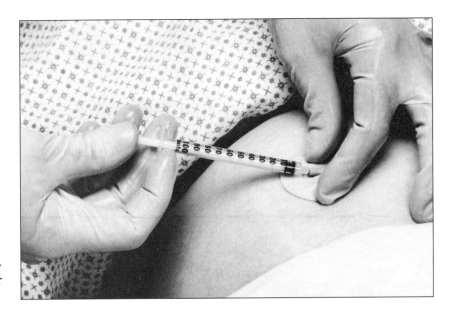

Removing the catheter

Take alcohol sponges, gloves, and an adhesive bandage to the patient's bedside. Explain the procedure to the patient, wash your hands, and put on gloves. Pull off the adhesive-backed foam disk at the insertion site.

▶ *Clinical tip:* To minimize the risk of infection, remove the used Insuflon catheter after inserting the new one.

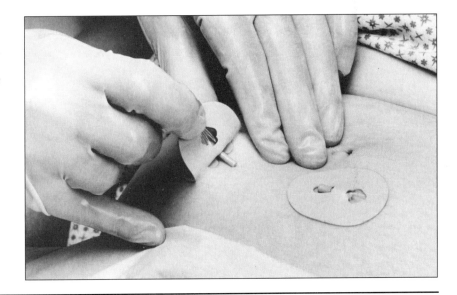

Holding on to the wings, remove the catheter with a gentle motion.

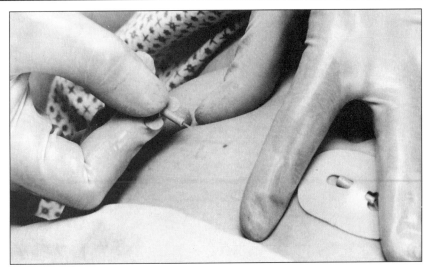

Next, wipe off any remaining adhesive with an alcohol sponge, and cover the site with an adhesive bandage. Document the procedure, the condition of the skin, and the patient's response in your nurse's notes.

 Clinical tip: To avoid problems with sticking and tangling, remove your gloves before you handle the adhesive bandage.

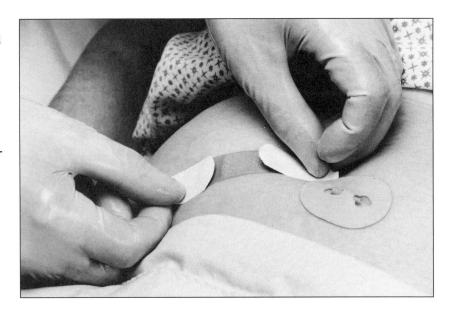

TROUBLESHOOTING

Solving problems related to the Insuflon catheter

PROBLEM	CAUSE	INTERVENTIONS
Meeting resistance when injecting insulin	Catheter obstruction	• Remove the catheter and insert a new one at a different site.
Redness, swelling, or pain	Infection at the insertion site	• Remove the catheter immediately and insert a new one at a different site. • Contact the doctor if symptoms continue for more than 24 hours.
Rash, itching, or eczema around the site	Allergic reaction to adhesive	• Obtain an order to apply 1% hydrocortisone cream. • If symptoms continue, try an alternative to ordinary adhesive tape (for example, hypoallergenic tape).
Elevated blood glucose level	Dead space in the catheter	• Obtain an order to add 0.5 unit of insulin to the first insulin injection after inserting a new catheter.
Accumulated condensate under the foam disk's protective transparent film	Trapped moisture	• Before applying a new foam disk, cut away part of the film around the catheter port.
Skin irritation	Discomfort from the plastic wings	• Place a thin piece of gauze under the wings before applying the foam pad.
Blood glucose level indicating a decreased response to insulin therapy or a lump or fatty cushion around the catheter tip	Lipohypertrophy	• Change the catheter site and remember to rotate the sites regularly. • Monitor the patient's blood glucose level closely. If it changes rapidly, contact the doctor, who may need to adjust the insulin dose.

GIVING INSULIN BY CONTINUOUS-INFUSION PUMP

Increasingly used by patients with insulin-dependent (Type I) diabetes mellitus, a subcutaneous continuous-infusion pump supplies long-term insulin therapy. This delivery system benefits patients who have widely fluctuating blood glucose levels despite compliance with drug and dietary regimens, those who don't eat regular meals, and those who are pregnant.

With a continuous-infusion pump, the patient can participate in therapy and may feel less anxiety because regular injections aren't necessary. What's more, the pump is relatively easy to use, which smoothes the transition from hospital to home for the patient and his family.

However, the continuous-infusion pump does have drawbacks, such as possible infection at the injection site, catheter clogging, and insulin loss from loose connections. Hyperglycemia and hypoglycemia may result if the pump is used incorrectly. Ketoacidosis may occur if the pump malfunctions.

UNDERSTANDING PUMP FEATURES

Various insulin infusion pumps are currently available. The MiniMed 506 pump, shown on the following pages, is about the size of a deck of cards and resembles a beeper. It's powered by three disposable batteries. Inside the pump, a syringe holds regular insulin, and a tiny computer controls syringe action by precisely regulating the insulin dosage.

The MiniMed 506 pump can be programmed to deliver insulin in bolus doses—the larger doses needed before meals and snacks—and in basal doses—the supplementary doses needed to maintain steady levels of insulin in the blood. (These basal doses, known as basal rates, and their associated delivery times are called *profiles*.) Once the pump is programmed, insulin from the syringe is delivered through an infusion set, composed of a catheter and an introducer needle, to a site under the patient's skin.

The pump has four buttons and a display screen. Pressing the appropriate buttons programs the pump. The SEL (select) button allows you to view the programming options. The ACT (activate) button initiates programming changes. The two arrow buttons allow you to program the pump precisely by scrolling through numerical values from high to low or from low to high.

The pump's syringe can be installed in two ways. In the short-syringe method, the syringe's neck stays almost completely concealed inside the pump. With this method, the syringe has a maximum volume of 150 units (U-100 insulin). In the full-syringe method, the luer-type neck of the syringe stays outside of the syringe compartment. This allows a maximum insulin volume of 300 units (U-100 insulin).

LOCATING INJECTION SITES

Appropriate insulin injection sites include the abdomen, upper hip, lower back, and thigh. These areas have ample subcutaneous tissue, so the patient feels minimal discomfort.

Preparing the pump

To begin using this pump, gather the necessary equipment: a MiniMed 506 pump, a Sof-set infusion set (designed for the pump), the MiniMed syringe (also designed for the pump), clean gloves, alcohol sponges, a 25G needle, insulin, and the patient's medication record.

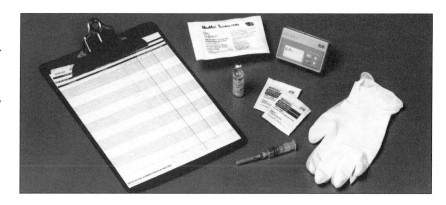

Pamela Kovach, RN, BSN, an independent nurse consultant for Springhouse Corporation, contributed to this section. The publisher thanks the following organizations for their help: *Advantage Health Services, Inc.,* Hatboro, Pa.; *MiniMed Technologies,* Sylmar, Calif.; and *Hill-Rom,* Batesville, Ind.

Take the equipment to the patient's bedside, explain the procedure, and compare the doctor's orders with the medication record. Wash your hands. Using sterile technique, attach the needle to the syringe. Insert the needle into the cap of the insulin vial, and fill the syringe with the ordered amount of insulin plus about 25 extra units to prime the infusion set.

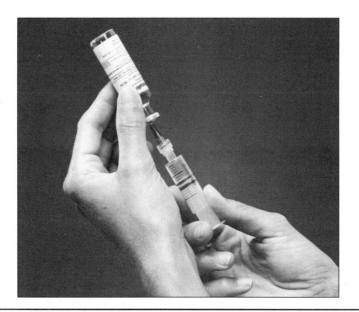

Remove and discard the needle. Next, connect the infusion set to the syringe, making sure that you tighten the connection between the infusion set and the syringe. Prime the infusion set by slowly advancing the plunger (as shown) until the infusion set fills and insulin drips from the needle at the end of the catheter.

▶ *Clinical tip:* To prevent a reduction in insulin delivery, make sure that you clear all air bubbles from the syringe and the infusion set.

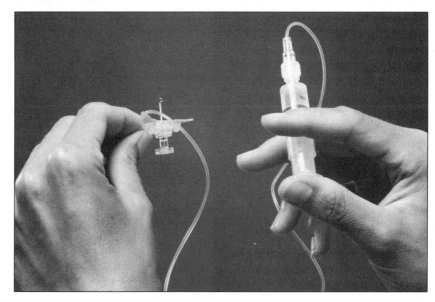

Installing the syringe

Depending on the drug volume ordered, you'll install the syringe in the pump by the short-syringe method (maximum volume 150 units of U-100 insulin) or the full-syringe method (maximum volume 300 units of U-100 insulin). To implement either method, first open the syringe compartment.

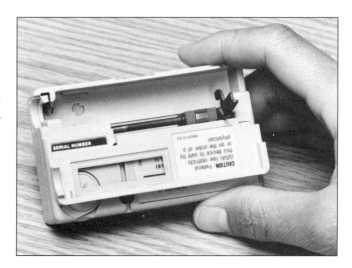

To use MiniMed's short-syringe method, first flip up the two driver arms. Slide them back as far as you can. Then flip up the silver luer-type neck holder. Insert the syringe by lining up its neck with the syringe converter. Firmly push down on the syringe. Then slide the two driver arms toward the syringe until they rest on each side of the plunger. Close the syringe compartment.

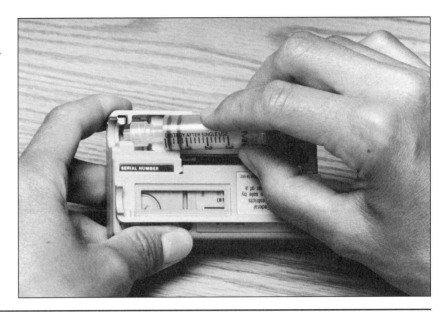

To use MiniMed's full-syringe method, first flip up the two driver arms. Slide them back as far as you can. Then flip up the silver luer-type neck holder. Insert the syringe by lining up its neck with the neck holder. Then push down on the syringe so that it fits firmly in place (as shown). Slide the two driver arms toward the syringe until they rest on each side of the syringe plunger. Close the compartment.

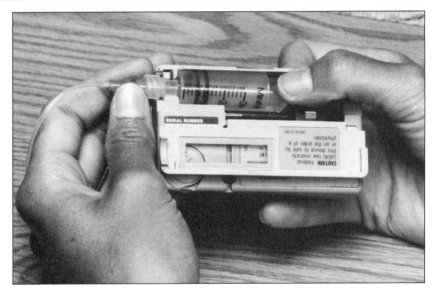

Testing the pump

To make sure that you've installed the syringe correctly, test the pump. Begin by setting the hour on the screen's clock display. To do this, press the ACT button. "SET HOURS" will appear on the screen. Then press the appropriate arrow buttons until you reach the correct hour. Be sure to set a.m. or p.m. Press the ACT button again to confirm the setting.

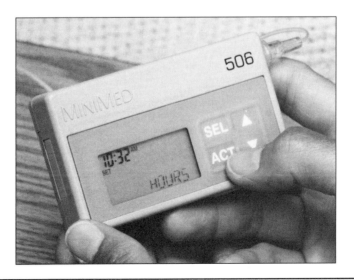

Now, set the minutes by pressing the ACT button. "SET MINUTES" will appear on the screen. Press the appropriate arrow buttons until you reach the correct number of minutes. Press the ACT button again to confirm the time.

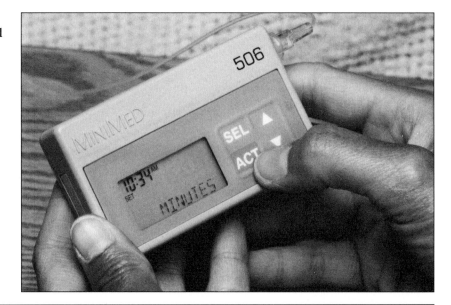

Next, set the day of the week. Start by pressing the ACT button. Then press the appropriate arrow buttons to select the correct day. Once you've done so, press ACT again.

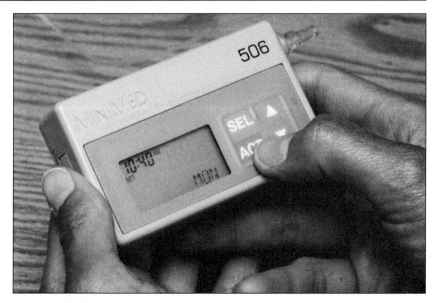

Finally, select the amount of insulin to be delivered. Press the SEL button and then the ACT button. The words "SET BOLUS" will appear. Use the arrow buttons to designate the ordered number of insulin units—in this case, 5 units. Press ACT again.

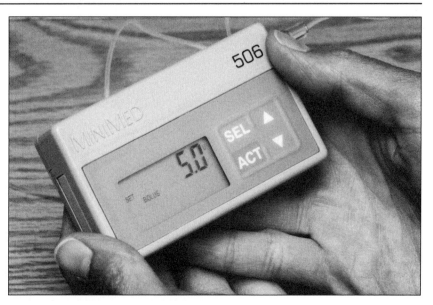

When you see insulin droplets appear at the needle tip, you know you've correctly inserted the syringe in the pump.

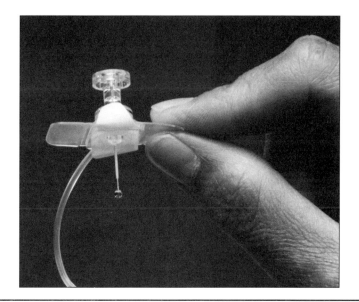

Starting the infusion

Before inserting the introducer needle, put on gloves. Choose the appropriate injection site, and clean it with an alcohol sponge or according to your hospital policy. Wipe in circles from the center outward. Let the site dry for at least 30 seconds.

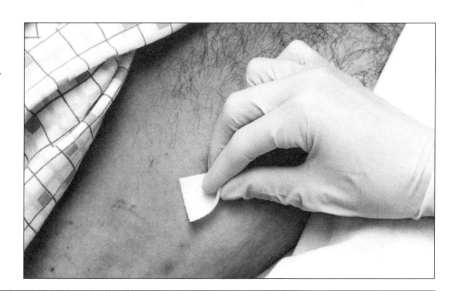

Remove the needle guard from the Sof-set infusion set, and pull off the white protective tab (as shown).

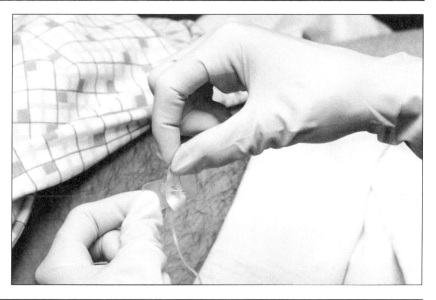

Hold the infusion set with your thumb and third finger. Put your index finger on top of the needle hub to stabilize it, and flex the wings upward (as shown). With your other hand, pinch the subcutaneous tissue as you would for giving an injection. Then quickly insert the needle at a 90-degree angle into the insertion site.

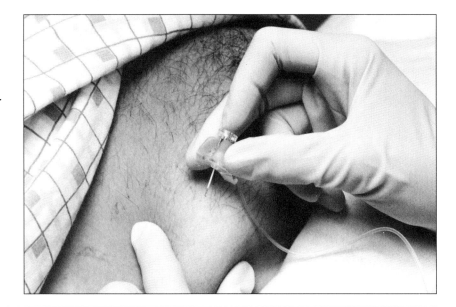

Peel off the white paper that lines the center of the Sof-set tape. Fit the hole in the tape over the needle hub, and apply the adhesive side of the tape over the Sof-set introducer needle. Pat the tape several times to secure it. Then peel off the paper liners at both ends of the tape, and smooth out the tape (as shown).

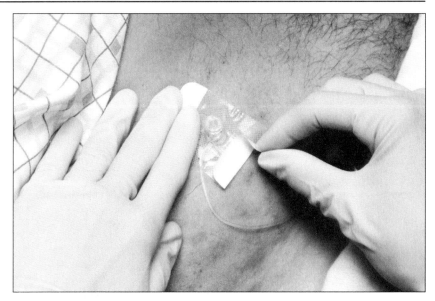

Next, remove the introducer needle from the insertion site. To do this, put the index and middle finger of one hand on each side of the Sof-set wings (as shown). Use your other hand to rotate the needle a half-turn. Then pull the introducer needle straight out.

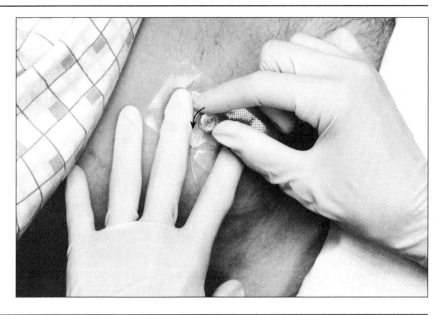

You may remove your gloves. Now set the bolus dose. Press the SEL button. The words "LAST BOLUS" should appear on the screen, along with the time and amount of the last bolus dose delivered. Continue by pressing ACT. "SET BOLUS" will appear on the screen (as shown). Press the arrow buttons to set the number of units to be delivered. Press the ACT button to activate the bolus and deliver the insulin.

Note: The pump beeps once when it finishes delivering the bolus dose; then the clock display reappears.

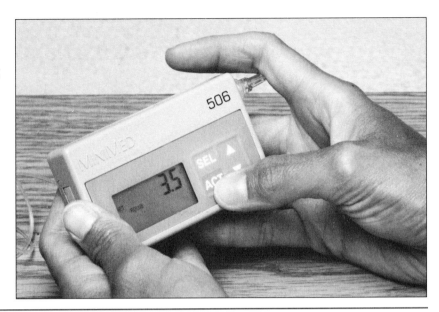

To set the basal dose and rate, press the SEL button three times and then press the ACT button. The screen will display the words "SET BASAL RATE PROFILE 1" and will show the time (12:00 a.m.). The words will blink, indicating that you can change the settings. Use the arrows to set the ordered basal rate for profile 1. Then press the ACT button. The pump will beep once to indicate that it has accepted the change.

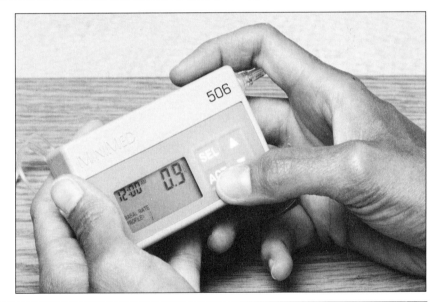

If you want to set only one profile, don't press any more buttons. The pump will automatically return to the clock display on the screen. To set multiple profiles, press the ACT button. The pump will beep once to indicate that it has accepted the change; then the screen will display "PROFILE 2." Use the arrow buttons to select another time and dose. Press the ACT button again. After you program all the profiles, the pump will automatically return to the clock display.

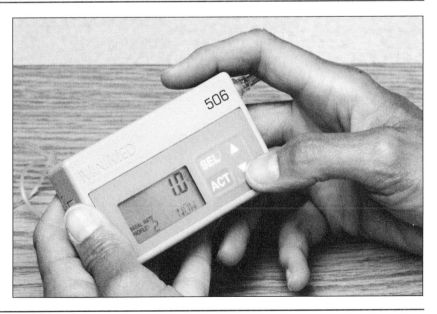

If you need to stop the infusion pump—to change the infusion set, for example—press the SEL button twice until the suspend display appears on the screen. Press ACT to stop the pump. The screen will display an "S" and the word "STOPPED," and the pump will stop (as shown). To restart the pump, press the SEL button, then the ACT button. The pump will beep, the clock display will reappear, and insulin delivery will resume.

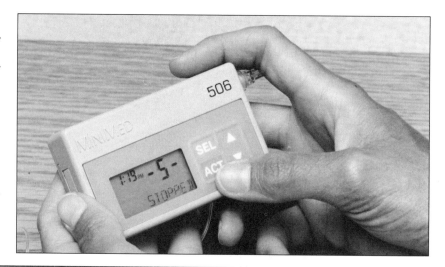

Finally, document the procedure on the patient's medication record. Record the amounts of the bolus dose and the basal doses (the profiles) along with the date, time, and injection site.

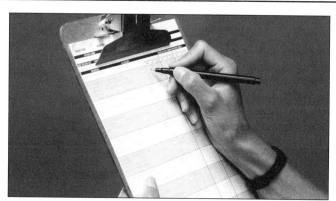

 TROUBLESHOOTING

Dealing with insulin pump problems

PROBLEM	POSSIBLE CAUSE	NURSING INTERVENTIONS
Clogged infusion set	• Unbuffered insulin • Poor site absorption • Very low basal rate • Infusion set left in place too long • Infusion set made of polyvinyl-chloride • Insulin inactivated because of temperature extremes	• Ask the doctor about using buffered insulin. • Change the infusion site. • Ask the doctor about further diluting insulin to increase the flow rate. • Change the set immediately, then regularly thereafter, following the manufacturer's instructions. • Use an infusion set made of polyolefin, which is more compatible with insulin. • Protect the pump and infusion set from temperature extremes. Change the infusion set, syringe, and insulin at the first sign of abnormal blood glucose levels.
Infusion site pain and irritation	• Infusion site changed too infrequently • Faulty insertion technique • Infusion site constricted	• Change the site as directed by hospital policy, the doctor, or both. • Use sterile technique to prevent infection and discomfort. • Change the site; don't start infusions in areas irritated by belts or tight clothing.
Blood in tubing	• Infusion site disturbed or jostled • Allergic reaction to needle	• Change the site and infusion set. • Ask the doctor about using a needleless infusion set.
Air bubbles in syringe	• Filling syringe with insulin	• After drawing the ordered amount of insulin, gently flick the syringe to remove bubbles.

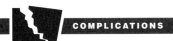

Correcting abnormal blood glucose levels with an infusion pump

Changes in food consumption, problems with the infusion pump, and other factors can contribute to abnormally high or low blood glucose levels. In some cases, you can correct these problems by adjusting the amount of insulin delivered by pump. Use this chart as a guide to possible causes of abnormal blood glucose levels and effective interventions.

BLOOD GLUCOSE LEVEL	POSSIBLE CAUSE	NURSING INTERVENTIONS
High More than 240 mg/dl on two consecutive readings	• Increased food intake • Bolus dose of insulin delivered too soon (or not at all) • Illness, stress, menses, or decreased exercise • Pump settings incorrectly programmed	• Reprogram insulin dosage as ordered. • Reprogram insulin bolus dose. • Reprogram insulin dosage as ordered. • Check pump settings, including bolus doses, profiles, insulin concentration, and total insulin delivered; reprogram settings as needed.
	• Empty syringe • Leaking infusion set or syringe • Air bubbles or obstruction in infusion set or syringe • Irritation at infusion site (redness, soreness, infection) • Unexplained	• Replace syringe. • Tighten the connection between the syringe and infusion set, or change the syringe and infusion set. • Change the infusion set and site. • Change the infusion set and site. • Test urine for ketone bodies. If test results are positive, call the doctor; if they're negative, change the infusion set.
Low Below 60 mg/dl	• Reduced food intake • Increased exercise or activity • Pump settings incorrectly programmed	• Reprogram insulin dosage as ordered. • Reprogram insulin dosage as ordered; decrease basal or bolus dose before exercise. • Check pump settings, including bolus doses, profiles, insulin concentration, and total insulin delivered; reprogram insulin settings as needed.
	• Infusion set incorrectly disconnected from syringe • Alcohol consumption in past 12 hours • Unexplained	• Review correct disconnection procedure to prevent excessive insulin infusion. • Check with doctor regarding hypoglycemic effect of alcohol. Reprogram insulin dosage as ordered. • Correct hypoglycemia. Reprogram insulin dosage as ordered. Monitor pump program settings.

GIVING AN INTRAMUSCULAR INJECTION

You'll give an intramuscular (I.M.) injection to deposit medication deep into muscle tissue that has a rich blood supply and allows rapid absorption into the systemic circulation. I.M. injections are recommended for patients who are uncooperative or who can't take medication orally and for drugs that are altered by digestive juices. Because muscle tissue has few sensory nerves, I.M. injection allows less painful administration of irritating drugs.

CHOOSING APPROPRIATE METHODS AND SITES

Choose the method and site of an I.M. injection carefully, taking into account your patient's general physical status, his age, and the purpose of the injection. (See *Locating I.M. injection sites.*)

The Z-track method of I.M. injection prevents leakage, or tracking, of injected medication into the subcutaneous (S.C.) tissue. You may need to use this method if your patient is elderly and has reduced muscle mass or if you're injecting an irritating medication. (See *Using the Z-track method,* page 100.)

Administration in adults and children

If your patient is a healthy adult, the gluteal muscles (gluteus medius, gluteus minimus, and the upper outer corner of the gluteus maximus) are the sites most commonly used. The deltoid muscle may be used for a small-volume injection (2 ml or less).

If your patient is an infant or a young child, however, the gluteal muscles are not appropriate. The rule of thumb in this age-group is the younger the child, the less developed the muscle. In a child under age 3 (or a child who hasn't been walking for at least 1 year), the gluteal muscles are not developed enough to receive an I.M. injection safely and without injury to the sciatic nerve. In this group, the thigh's vastus lateralis muscle is the most common site for an I.M. injection because it's usually better developed than the gluteal muscles and has no large nerves or blood vessels. These factors minimize the risk of injury. Other appropriate sites are the deltoid muscle (in children), if it's sufficiently developed, and the rectus femoris muscle (in infants).

Administration in elderly patients

An elderly patient usually has less S.C. tissue and less muscle mass (especially in the buttocks and del-

toid muscles), so you may need to use a shorter needle. Also, an elderly patient typically has more fat around the hips, abdomen, and thighs. This makes the vastus lateralis muscle and ventrogluteal area (gluteus medius and minimus, but not gluteus maximus muscles) primary injection sites. If the patient is extremely thin, pinch the muscle gently to elevate it and to avoid putting the needle completely through the muscle. Never give an I.M. injection in an immobile limb because of poor drug absorption and the risk of sterile abscess.

Because of age-related vascular changes, elderly patients are also at greater risk for hematomas. To control bleeding, you may need to apply direct pressure over the puncture site for longer than usual. Gently massage the injection site to aid drug absorption and distribution. However, avoid site massage with certain drugs given using the Z-track method, such as iron dextran or hydroxyzine hydrochloride.

REPEATING INJECTIONS

Rotate the injection sites if your patient requires repeated injections. Also remember that I.M. injections require sterile technique to maintain the integrity of muscle tissue. The prescribed medication also must be sterile. The needle may be packaged separately or already attached to the syringe. Needles used for I.M. injections are longer than those used for S.C. injections because they must reach deep into the muscle. Needle length depends on the injection site, the patient's size, and the amount of fat covering the muscle. The needle gauge for I.M. injections should be larger than that used for S.C. injections to accommodate viscous solutions and suspensions.

REVIEWING CONTRAINDICATIONS

Avoid administering I.M. injections at inflamed, edematous, or irritated sites or at sites with moles, birthmarks, scar tissue, or other lesions. I.M. injections may also be contraindicated in patients with impaired coagulation mechanisms and in those with conditions that impair peripheral absorption, such as peripheral vascular disease and shock.

Locating I.M. injection sites

Once you've selected the deltoid, ventrogluteal, dorsogluteal, or vastus lateralis muscle for an I.M. injection, you'll need to locate the specific needle insertion site (dotted areas) and choose the proper needle angle.

Deltoid

To locate the deltoid muscle, find the lower edge of the acromial process and the point on the lateral arm in line with the axilla. Insert the needle 1″ to 2″ (2.5 to 5 cm) below the acromial process (usually two to three fingerbreadths) at a 90-degree angle or at an angle slightly toward the process.

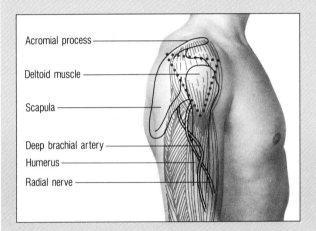

Dorsogluteal

You'll give a dorsogluteal injection above and outside a line drawn from the posterior superior iliac spine to the greater trochanter of the femur. Or divide the buttock into quadrants and inject into the upper outer quadrant, about 2″ to 3″ (5 to 8 cm) below the iliac crest. Insert the needle at a 90-degree angle.

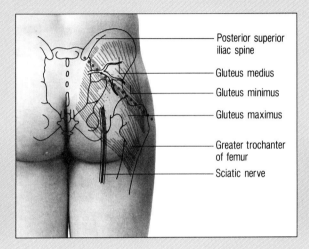

Ventrogluteal

To give a ventrogluteal injection, locate the greater trochanter of the femur with the heel of your hand. Then spread your index and middle fingers from the anterior superior iliac spine to as far along the iliac crest as you can reach. Insert the needle between the two fingers at a 90-degree angle to the muscle. (Remove your hand before inserting the needle.)

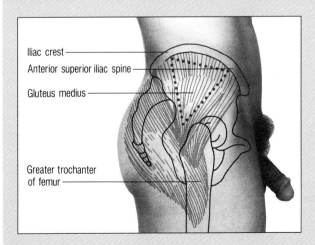

Vastus lateralis

Use the vastus lateralis—the lateral muscle of the quadriceps group—from a handbreadth below the greater trochanter to a handbreadth above the knee. Insert the needle into the middle third of the muscle parallel to the surface on which your patient lies. You may have to bunch the muscle before insertion.

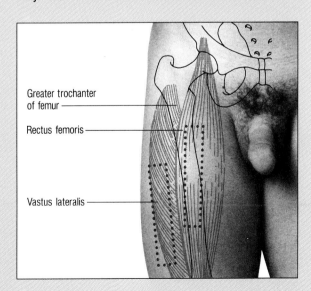

Using the Z-track method

If you're administering an irritating drug, such as iron dextran, or giving an injection to an elderly patient with decreased muscle mass, you'll need to vary the standard I.M. procedure by using the Z-track method. By staggering the needle pathway after injection, this technique allows I.M. drug delivery while minimizing the risk of subcutaneous staining and irritation from certain drugs. You'll inject the drug into the patient's buttock. But never inject more than 5 ml into a single site using this method. The illustrations below show you how to perform a Z-track injection. Before the procedure begins, the skin, subcutaneous fat, fascia, and muscle lie in their normal positions, as shown.

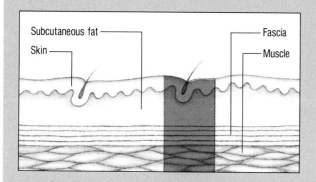

After drawing up 0.3 to 0.5 cc of air into the syringe, replace the needle with a sterile one that's 3″ (8 cm) long. Put on gloves. Then place your finger on the skin surface, and pull the skin and subcutaneous layers out of alignment with the underlying muscle (see below). Move the skin about 1″ (2.5 cm). This ensures entry of the injected medication into the muscle tissue.

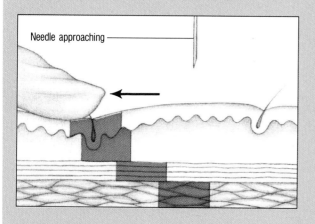

After cleaning the site, insert the needle at a 90-degree angle in the site where you initially placed your finger (see below). Inject the drug slowly. When the injection is complete, wait 10 seconds before withdrawing the needle. This keeps the medication from seeping out of the injection site.

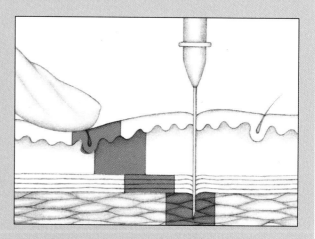

After withdrawing the needle, allow the retracted skin to resume its normal position. The needle track (shown by the broken line) is now broken at the junction of each tissue layer, trapping the drug in the muscle.

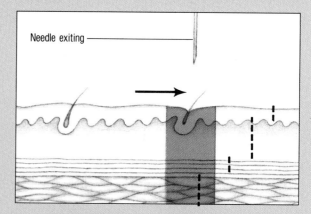

Never massage the site or allow the patient to wear a tight-fitting garment over the site. Either action could force the medication into the subcutaneous tissue and cause irritation. To increase the rate of absorption, encourage physical activity such as walking. For subsequent injections, alternate buttocks.

Begin by gathering the necessary equipment: the prescribed medication, the patient's medication record, a 3- to 5-ml syringe, a 20G to 25G 1″ to 3″ needle, gloves, and alcohol sponges.

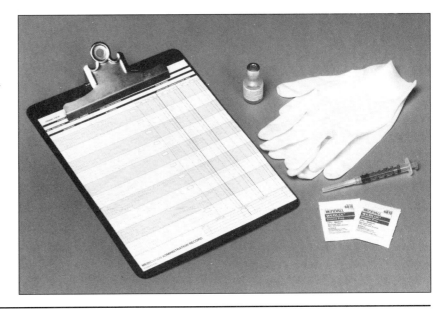

Verify the order on the patient's medication record by checking it against the doctor's order. Also check the patient's allergy history and verify his identity. Inspect the prescribed drug for color, clarity, and expiration date. Never use an expired, cloudy, or precipitous solution unless the manufacturer's instructions allow it. Remember also that some drugs (such as suspensions) normally contain particles. Then provide privacy and explain the procedure to the patient. Position and drape him appropriately, making sure that the injection site is well lighted and exposed (as shown). Put on gloves.

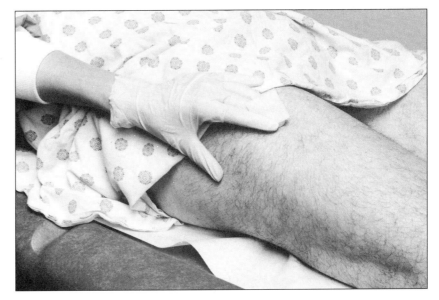

Loosen the protective needle sheath, but don't remove it. After selecting the injection site, gently tap it to stimulate nerve endings and minimize pain when you insert the needle.

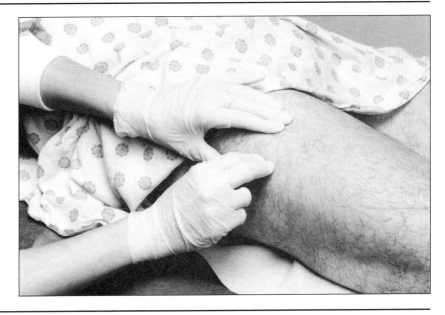

Next, clean the skin at the site with an alcohol sponge. Move the sponge outward in a circular motion to a circumference of about 2″ (5 cm) from the injection site. Allow the skin to dry to avoid introducing alcohol into the needle puncture, which causes pain.

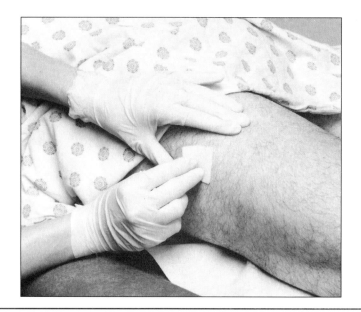

With the thumb and index finger of your nondominant hand, gently stretch the skin taut at the injection site.

▶ *Clinical tip:* Always encourage the patient to relax the muscle you'll be injecting because injections into tense muscles are more painful and cause more bleeding.

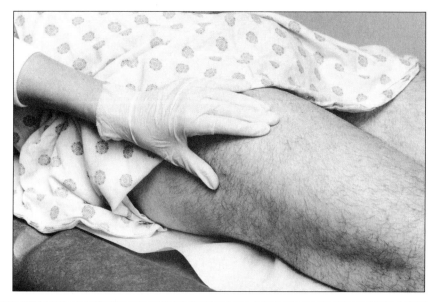

Holding the syringe in your dominant hand, remove the needle sheath by slipping it between the free fingers of your nondominant hand and then drawing back the syringe. Position the syringe at a 90-degree angle to the skin surface, with the needle a couple of inches from the skin. Tell the patient that he'll feel a prick as you insert the needle. Then quickly and firmly thrust the needle through the skin and S.C. tissue, deeply into the muscle.

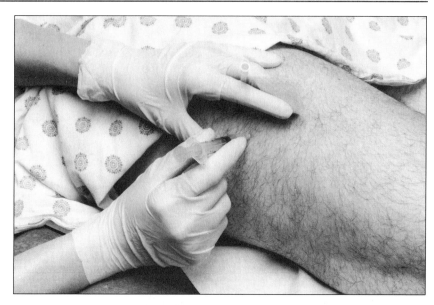

Because you won't recap the needle, discard the cap. Then support the syringe with your nondominant hand if desired (as shown). Pull back slightly on the plunger with your dominant hand to aspirate for blood. If blood appears in the syringe on aspiration, you'll know that the needle is in a blood vessel. In such a case, stop the injection and withdraw the needle. Don't inject the bloody solution. Instead, prepare another injection with new equipment and use another injection site.

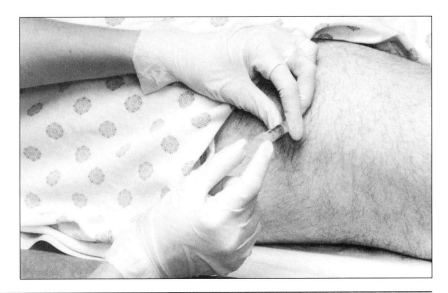

If no blood appears in the syringe, proceed. Place your thumb on the plunger rod. Slowly and steadily inject the medication into the muscle, allowing the muscle to distend gradually and accept the medication under minimal pressure. You should feel little or no resistance against the force of the injection.

▶ **Clinical tip:** If the patient experiences pain or anxiety with repeated injections, use ice to numb the area before cleaning. Hold the ice in place for several seconds. If you must inject more than 5 ml of solution, divide the solution and inject it at two separate sites.

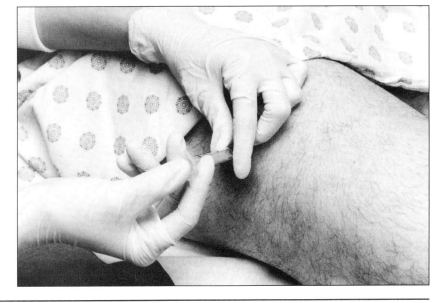

After the injection, gently but quickly remove the needle at a 90-degree angle. Using a gloved hand, cover the injection site immediately with an alcohol sponge (as shown). Apply gentle pressure and, unless contraindicated, massage the relaxed muscle to help distribute the drug and promote absorption. Remove the alcohol sponge, and inspect the injection site for signs of active bleeding or bruising. If bleeding continues, apply pressure to the site; if bruising occurs, you may apply ice. Watch for adverse reactions at the site for 30 minutes after the injection. Discard all equipment according to hospital policy.

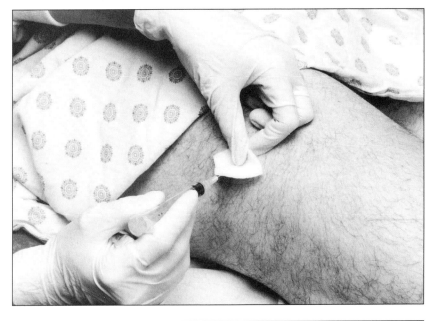

Giving I.M. injections to infants and toddlers

Generally, you'll adapt the principles of adult I.M. administration for children, basing changes on the differences in muscle mass between adults and children. Use a 25G to 27G ½″ to 1″ needle. The volume injected should not exceed 0.5 ml in an infant or 1 ml in a small child. Another important difference involves the need to restrain any child under age 5 during an I.M. injection. If you're using the anterior thigh (vastus lateralis), position the child as shown. Grasp the chosen leg firmly below the knee with your nondominant hand. Lean across the child's torso with your upper body, being careful not to put too much pressure on the child's chest. With your dominant hand, administer the injection.

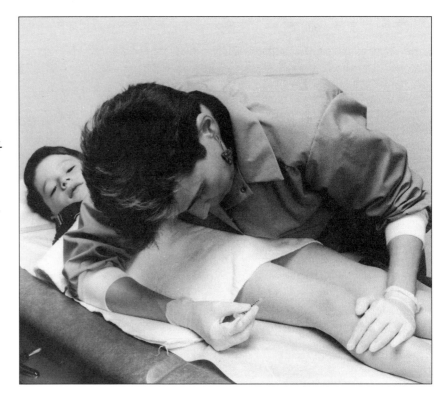

GIVING A NEEDLE-FREE INJECTION

Needle-stick injuries put health care workers at risk for infection, especially with hepatitis B and human immunodeficiency virus (HIV). Today, however, the risk can be eliminated by using a device such as the Biojector 2000, featured on the following pages, which delivers medication without a needle.

This injector uses carbon dioxide (CO_2) to drive a plunger that propels medication through a microorifice and into subcutaneous tissue or muscle.

The CO_2 never comes in contact with the medication. And each dose of medication is given with a separate sterile syringe, eliminating the risk of cross-contamination among patients.

Most commonly injected drugs can be administered with the needle-free injector. To maximize drug effectiveness and patient comfort, you'll need to select the right size syringe for the site and tissue to be used (see *Choosing the right injector syringe*).

Choosing the right injector syringe

When using a needle-free injection system, be sure to select a syringe designed for the drug administration route and site and the patient's body type. Use this chart as a guide.

SYRINGE # AND COLOR	ROUTE	INJECTION SITE	BODY TYPE
No. 2 green	S.C.	All standard S.C. sites	All patients
No. 3 brown	I.M.	• Thigh • Deltoid	• Height, 15" to 20" (38 to 51 cm); weight, 0 to 15 lb (0 to 7 kg) • Height, 21" to 47" (53 to 119 cm); weight, 16 to 50 lb (7.3 to 23 kg)
No. 4 blue	I.M.	• Thigh or gluteus • Deltoid	• Height, 21" to 47" (53 to 119 cm); weight, 16 to 75 lb (7.3 to 34 kg) • Small adults (weighing less than 80% of lean body weight for their height) and children over 50 lb
No. 5 silver	I.M.	Deltoid	Adults of average body size (within 20% of lean body weight for their height)
No. 7 red	I.M.	Deltoid	Large adults (weighing more than 120% of lean body weight for their height)

Karen E. Michael, RN, MSN, a case manager with Greater Atlantic Health Service in Philadelphia, contributed to this section. The publisher thanks *Hill-Rom,* Batesville, Ind., and *Bioject Inc.,* Portland, Ore., for their help.

To use this needle-free injector system, you'll need the Biojector injector.

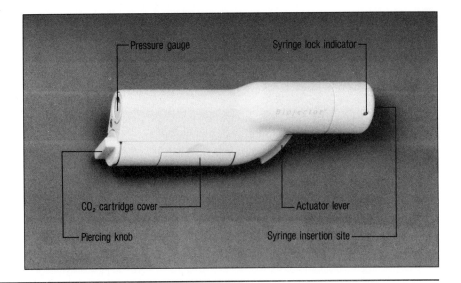

You'll also need a Bioject syringe device (which contains a disposable syringe and a fill tube with needle), a special syringe cap, a CO_2 cartridge, a vial of the prescribed medication, gloves, alcohol sponges, several $3'' \times 3''$ gauze pads, and an adhesive bandage.

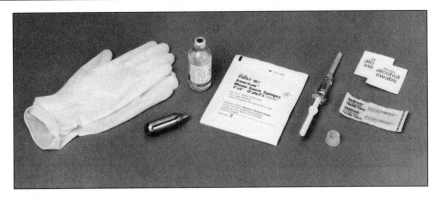

Take the equipment to the patient's bedside. Then wash your hands. Explain the procedure to the patient and tell her that local reactions (such as skin irritation, induration, bleeding, and ecchymosis) may occur at the injection site, just as they may with a syringe and needle.

Verify the medication order in the patient's chart, and then check the indicator needle on the pressure gauge at the rear of the injector. The needle should rest in the positive (green) section of the pressure gauge (as shown).

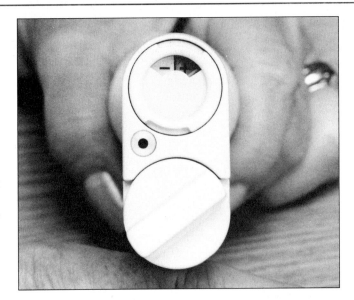

Unloading and reloading the CO₂ cartridge

If the indicator needle is in the center or the negative (white) area rather than the positive area, replace the CO_2 cartridge.

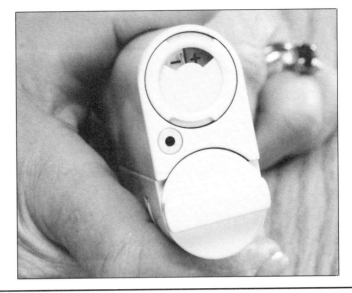

To do this, turn the cartridge piercing knob counterclockwise as far as it will go (near right). You may hear the sound of residual CO_2 being released.

To remove the cartridge, hold the injector device with the cartridge compartment facing up. Open the cartridge cover, push the cartridge forward slightly, tip the injector down, let the cartridge fall out (far right), and discard it.

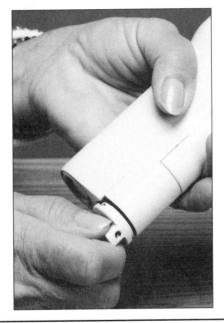
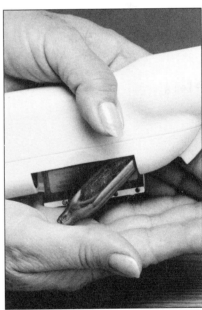

Insert the new CO_2 cartridge into the chamber by pushing the large end gently forward into the chamber and then gently pushing the small end into the chamber so that the small end faces the rear of the device.

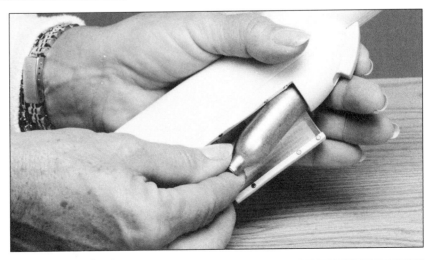

Close the cartridge cover and turn the piercing knob clockwise. When you meet resistance, quickly tighten the piercing knob. You may hear the sound of CO_2 filling the injector device. Then check the pressure gauge to ensure that the indicator needle is in the positive area.

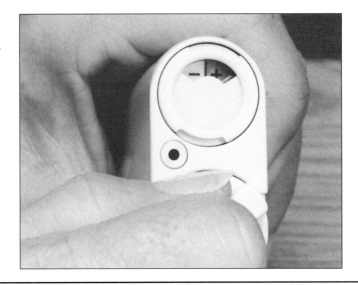

Filling the syringe

Carefully open the syringe package and remove the syringe assembly and the safety cap. Next, remove the protective cover from the fill needle. Draw the prescribed medication from the vial into the syringe, just as you would if you were using a standard syringe. Don't fill the syringe beyond the 1-ml line.

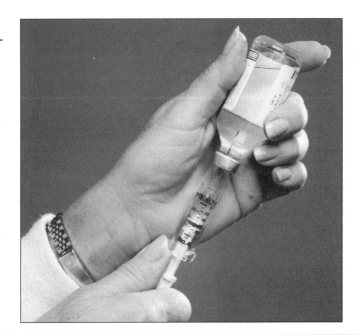

Once the medication is in the syringe, replace the needle cover. Do so by using the one-handed technique approved by the Centers for Disease Control and Prevention (as shown). Remove the needle from the syringe, and discard the needle properly in a sharps container.

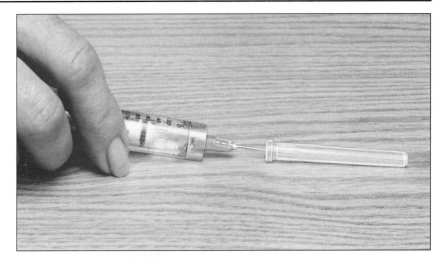

To avoid touching and contaminating the syringe, put the protective cap over the tip of the medication syringe. Do this by placing the cap on a firm, level surface and lowering the syringe barrel into the cap.

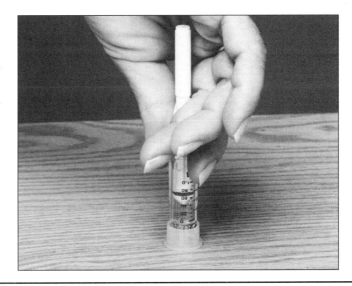

Inserting the syringe

Insert the filled syringe into the injector (near right), aligning the notches in the top of the syringe barrel with the matching grooves in the collar of the device. Turn the syringe about one-quarter turn clockwise to lock it in place. Then check the syringe lock indicator to make sure that green appears in the window (far right).

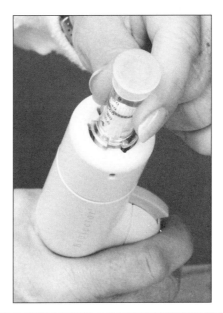
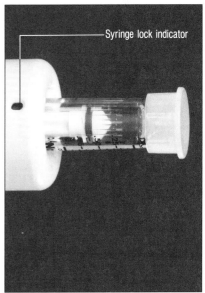

Syringe lock indicator

Injecting the medication

Put on gloves and clean the injection site on the patient's skin with an alcohol sponge. Using a circular motion, wipe from the center of the site outward.

▶ *Clinical tip:* Make sure that you allow sufficient time for the skin to dry. If it isn't dry when you inject the drug, the patient may feel a sting from the alcohol. Or the moisture may cause the syringe tip to slide and possibly lacerate the skin.

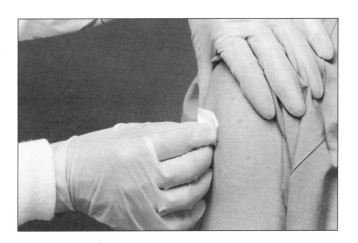

Hold the patient's skin firmly enough to prevent skin movement during the injection. Position the injector at a 90-degree angle to the skin, and press the device firmly into the skin to ensure that the medication penetrates with as little discomfort for the patient as possible.

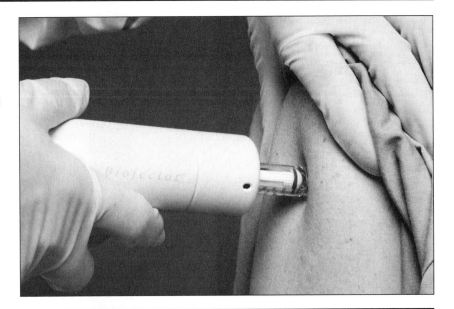

Remind the patient to relax her muscle. To administer the medication, press and release the actuator lever (on the underside of the injector device) in one slow, smooth motion. You may hear a hissing sound when you do so. This is the normal sound of CO_2 escaping from the device.

▶ *Clinical tip:* Do not move the injector while delivering the medication; hold it in place for 1 or 2 seconds after delivering the medication.

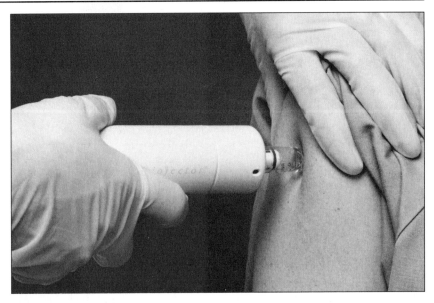

Remove the injector device. Using a 3″ × 3″ gauze pad, apply pressure to the site for about 1 minute (near right) to minimize bleeding and reduce the possibility of infection. Apply an adhesive bandage to the site. Then remove the syringe from the injector (far right), and dispose of it in the proper medical waste container.

Wash your hands and document the procedure in the medical record (include the name of the medication, the injection site, the time and date of the injection, and the patient's response).

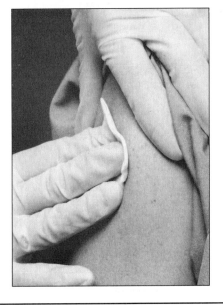 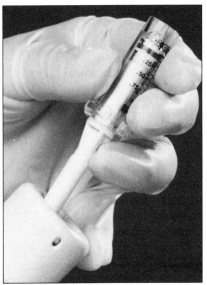

USING A RETRACTABLE NEEDLE AND SYRINGE

How many close calls or actual needle sticks have you had after administering an injection? Even one is too many. Fortunately, new devices are available to help you avoid injury. One of them—the SafeSnap retractable needle syringe—is described here. This system retracts the used needle into the barrel of the syringe, shielding you from accidental contact with the needle and preventing reuse of the needle. Syringes are available in 1-ml, 3-ml, 5-ml, and 10-ml sizes.

To use the SafeSnap system, gather the following equipment and take it to the patient's bedside: the right size SafeSnap syringe, the prescribed medication, gloves, and alcohol sponges.

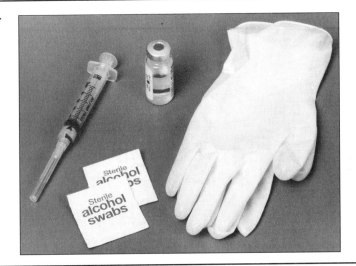

Check the medication order in the patient's medical record, and confirm the patient's identification on his hospital bracelet. Explain the procedure, wash your hands, and draw up the correct amount of medication in the syringe.

▶ *Clinical tip:* Make sure that the clip, which is red, is in the locked position to prevent the needle from retracting into the barrel before the injection.

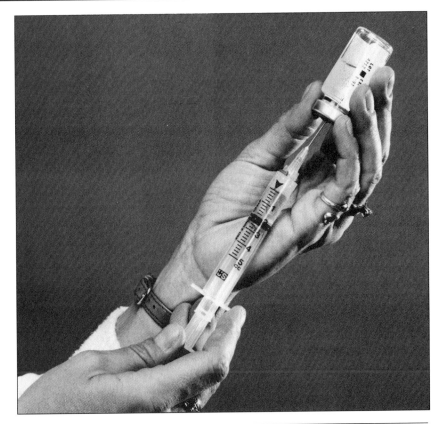

Karen E. Michael, RN, MSN, a case manager with Greater Atlantic Health Service in Philadelphia, contributed to this section. The publisher thanks *Hill-Rom,* Batesville, Ind., and *U.S. Medical Instruments, Inc.,* San Diego, Calif., for their help.

Put on gloves. Then use an alcohol sponge to clean the injection site. Let the area dry; then administer the medication by the prescribed route, using the appropriate technique.

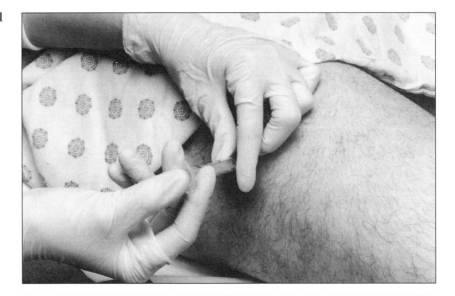

Push the plunger in as far as it will go until it clicks into the needle. Then remove the needle from the patient. The plunger will be locked into place as shown.

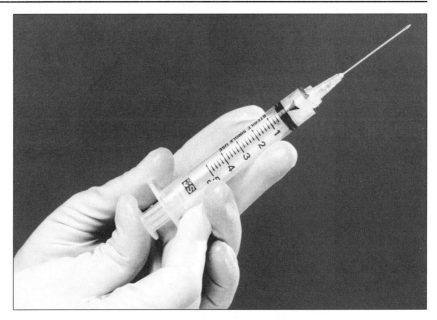

Flip open the clip near the hub of the syringe.

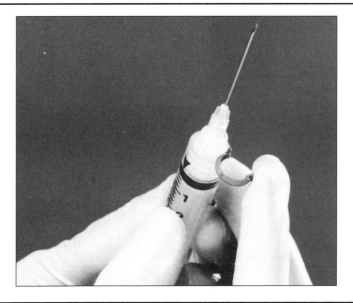

Next, pull the plunger to draw the needle all the way into the barrel. ▶ *Clinical tip:* You can flip the clip while the needle is still in the patient. Do this by grasping the syringe and pulling back the plunger after you inject the medication. The needle will completely retract into the barrel.

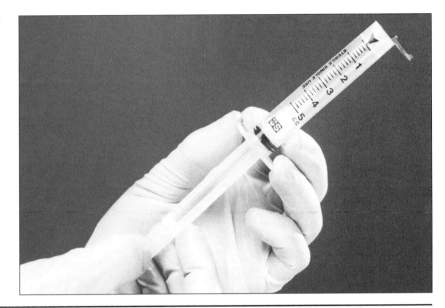

Break the plunger off with a quick snapping motion.

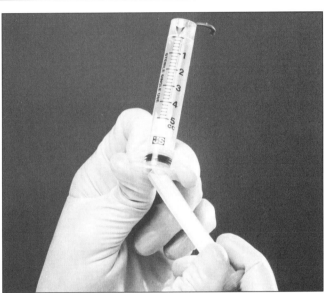

Insert the plunger into the open end of the barrel.

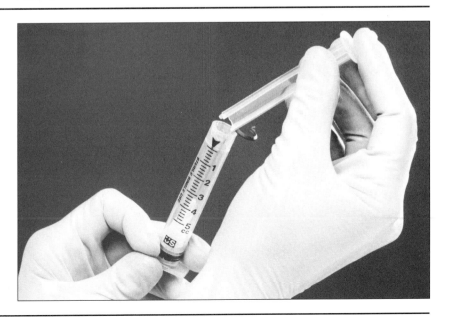

Continue to push the plunger into the barrel until you hear a click.

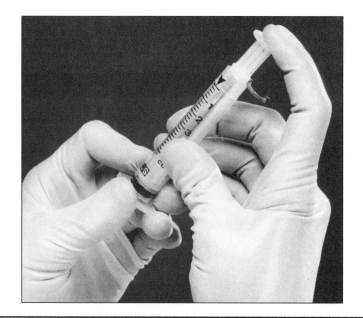

Dispose of the barrel and needle assembly in the appropriate container according to your hospital's policy. Remove your gloves and wash your hands. Document the procedure and the patient's response.

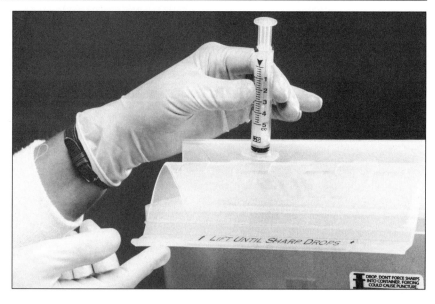

INFUSING DRUGS THROUGH A SECONDARY I.V. LINE

A secondary I.V. line is used for continuous or intermittent infusion. It connects to the Y-port of the patient's primary I.V. line rather than directly to the venipuncture device. When the secondary setup delivers solution intermittently, it's known as a *piggyback infusion*. When it supplies a solution continuously over several hours, it's known as a *continuous secondary I.V. infusion*. A complete setup for a secondary I.V. line includes a solution container, tubing, and a microdrip or macrodrip system.

With a piggyback infusion, the primary I.V. line maintains venous access between drug doses. When using this setup, you'll need to assemble a small (25- to 250-ml) I.V. container, short I.V. tubing, and a macrodrip system. Then you'll connect the setup to the upper Y-port (known as the piggyback port) of the primary I.V. line.

The primary I.V. line usually contains a piggyback port with a backcheck valve that stops the flow from the primary line during secondary drug infusion and returns the flow to the primary line after secondary drug infusion. Histamine$_2$-receptor antagonists and antibiotics are the agents most commonly administered by piggyback infusion.

With a continuous secondary I.V. infusion, you'll set up longer, full-length I.V. tubing and connect it to the lower Y-port of the primary I.V. line. This secondary line permits drug infusion and titration while the primary line maintains a constant total infusion rate.

A secondary I.V. line poses certain risks even when it's set up with meticulous care. For example, repeatedly introducing a needle into the port will increase the chance of contaminating the tubing. And administering a dose from the secondary line into the primary line can cause problems if drugs or other solutions are incompatible. To safeguard your patient, make sure that he already has a primary I.V. line with a Y-port. Then match the order on the patient's medication record with the doctor's order. Also confirm that the secondary I.V. solution and medication are compatible with the solution in the patient's primary I.V. line.

Preparing a secondary line

To set up a secondary I.V. line, gather these supplies: the prescribed I.V. medication (usually premixed in a minibag), continuous secondary tubing or piggyback extension tubing, an extension hook, a 20G (or smaller) 1″ needle, a medication label (if you're not using a premixed solution), alcohol sponges, 1″ adhesive tape, and the patient's medication and intake and output records (as shown).

If the solutions and medications are incompatible, you'll also need two 3-ml syringes (filled with 0.9% sodium chloride solution) and a 22G 1″ needle. You may also need an infusion pump or time tape. Usually the medication is prepared in a medication area.

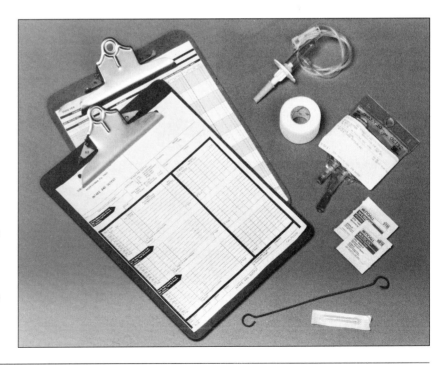

Contributors to this section include *Mary Jane McDevitt, RN, BS*, an oncology nurse at Mercy Catholic Medical Center, Fitzgerald Mercy Division, Darby, Pa., and *Denise Salvo, RN,C, MSN, CCRN*, an instructor at Widener University, Chester, Pa. The publisher thanks the following organizations for their help: *Baxter Healthcare Corp., Edwards Critical-Care Division*, Irvine, Calif.; *Doylestown (Pa.) Hospital;* and *Hill-Rom*, Batesville, Ind.

Next, wash your hands. Obtain or prepare the medication for infusion. Depending on hospital policy, I.V. medications may be premixed by the pharmacy or prepared by the nurse. In either case, verify that the medication you're using is the one that the doctor ordered. Compare the label on the medication container with the order on the medication record.

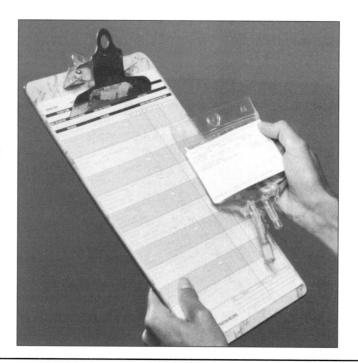

If you need to add a medication to a secondary I.V. solution, remove any seals from the secondary container. (In general, I.V. solution bags have a sealed outlet and an unsealed injection port, whereas bottled solutions have a seal covering their dual-outlet port.) Clean the injection port with an alcohol sponge. Inject the prescribed medication, and gently agitate the solution to mix the medication thoroughly. Label the I.V. mixture with the patient's name; the date; the drug name, amount, and dosage; and your initials.

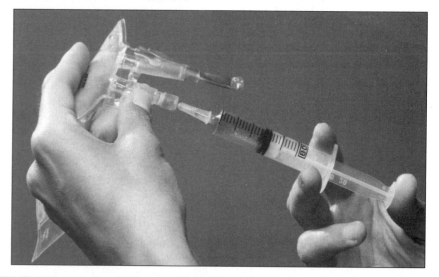

Remove the secondary administration set from its packaging. Straighten the tubing and close the roller clamp. Remove the protective cap from the distal end of the tubing, and attach the 20G (or smaller) needle.

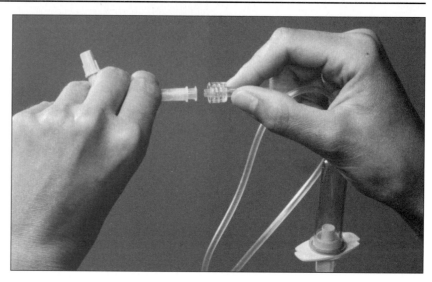

Remove the protective cap from the infusion (outlet) port of the I.V. medication bag; then remove the cap from the I.V. tubing spike. Insert the spike into the port of the I.V. medication bag.

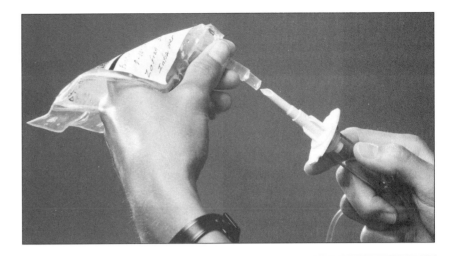

Hang the bag on an I.V. pole. Squeeze the drip chamber of the I.V. tubing, and allow the chamber to fill halfway.

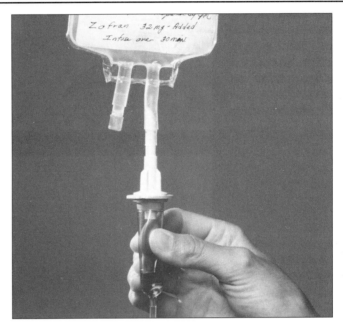

Open the roller clamp and prime the I.V. tubing and needle by allowing the solution to flow through it (as shown). Close the roller clamp when the solution reaches the tip of the needle.

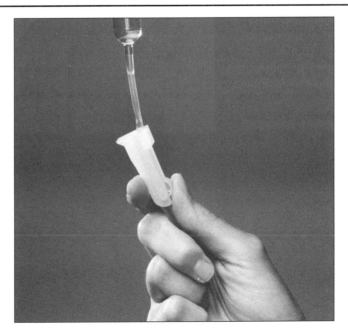

If you haven't already done so, take the equipment and the prepared I.V. solution to the patient's bedside. Examine the primary I.V. container for cracks or leaks. Examine the primary line to locate the Y-port. For a piggyback infusion, the port should lie above the roller clamp (as shown). For a continuous secondary infusion, it should be near the lower end of the primary line.

▶ *Clinical tip:* If you're administering a piggyback infusion, make sure that the primary line also has a backcheck valve, either above the upper Y-port or in the Y-port itself. If the tubing doesn't have a backcheck valve and you'll be infusing medication regularly, substitute tubing that has a backcheck valve.

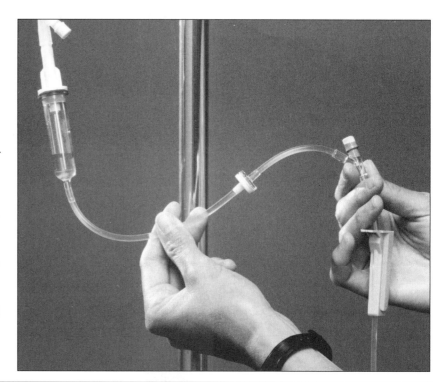

Starting the secondary infusion

Ask the patient his name. Then compare the name, room number, and bed number on his identification bracelet with the same information on the medication record. Tell the patient what the medication is and describe the procedure to him.

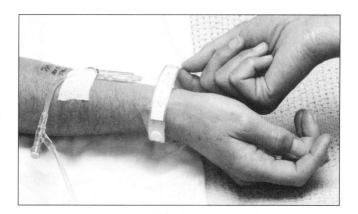

Providing a piggyback infusion

Hang the piggyback setup on the I.V. pole. Using an alcohol sponge, clean the Y-port above the roller clamp of the primary I.V. tubing. Insert the needle from the piggyback line into the Y-port of the primary line.

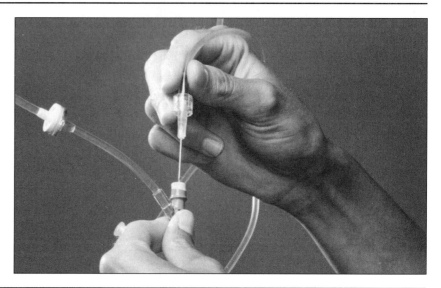

Tape this connection securely
(near right), unless you're using a
recessed needle, which doesn't require taping. Instead, a plastic covering may lock the needle in place
(far right).
▶ **Clinical tip:** To reduce the
risk of needle-stick injury,
use a needleless system or a click-
lock system with any type of secondary infusion or with an intermittent infusion device.

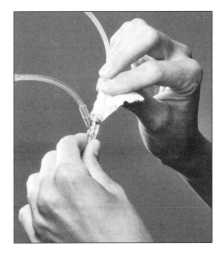 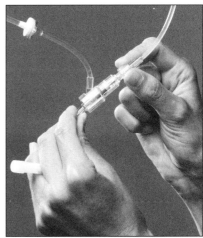

To infuse the piggyback medication without infusing the fluid
from the primary I.V. bag or bottle, hang the primary I.V. bag or
bottle below the level of the piggyback container. Use the extension
hook supplied with the piggyback
infusion set. To infuse the primary and secondary solutions si-
multaneously, hang them at the
same height.

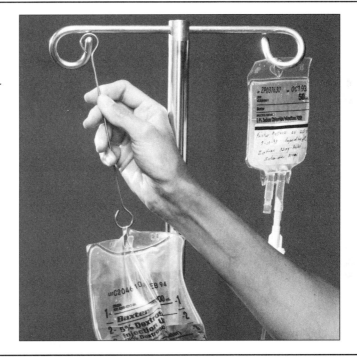

Completely open the roller clamp
on the piggyback tubing. Then adjust the roller clamp of the primary set to regulate the infusion
rate of the piggyback infusion.
The primary I.V. solution won't run
while the piggyback medication is
infusing. If the secondary I.V. solution isn't compatible with the primary I.V. solution, be sure to flush
the primary line before and after
infusing the incompatible solution.

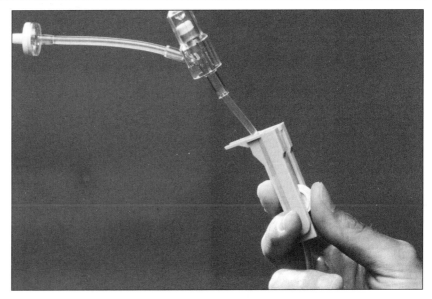

Providing a continuous secondary infusion

If you're administering a continuous secondary infusion, adjust the roller clamp on the tubing of the secondary solution to the desired drip rate. Then adjust the roller clamp on the tubing of the primary solution to achieve the desired total infusion rate.

▶ *Clinical tip:* If your hospital policy allows, use a pump or a time tape on the secondary line to maintain an even flow rate.

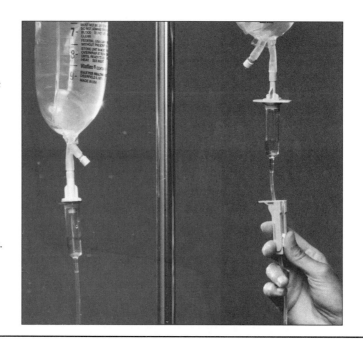

If you're using a continuous secondary setup and the primary and secondary solutions are incompatible, stop the primary infusion. Before beginning the secondary infusion, flush the line with 2 or 3 ml of 0.9% sodium chloride solution (as shown). Then administer the secondary infusion. Once you complete the secondary infusion, flush the line again before resuming the primary infusion. If you can't interrupt the primary infusion, use a double-lumen catheter, or administer the medication through another I.V. site.

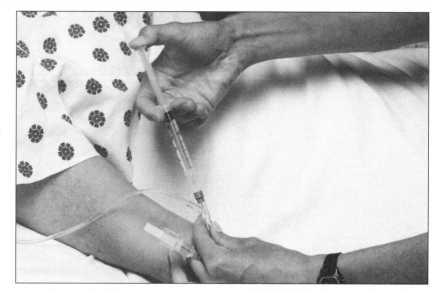

Adding a T-connector to the line

One way to resolve incompatibility problems is to use a T-connector. This device allows simultaneous administration of drugs and fluids or of a primary I.V. solution and an incompatible drug. A T-connector is a 3″ to 6″ (8- to 15-cm) piece of small-bore extension tubing fitted with an injection port near the luer-lock connection and a slide clamp. To attach the T-connector to the tubing, you'll need tape and gloves (because you'll be manipulating the hub of the venipuncture device).

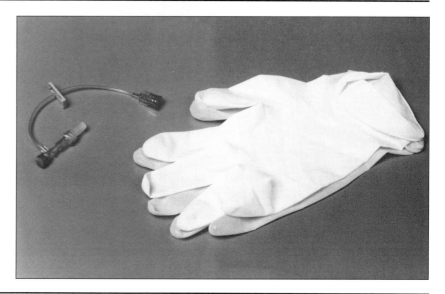

Wash your hands and put on gloves to protect you from possible contact with body fluids. Explain the procedure to the patient. Prime the T-connector tubing with I.V. fluid. Then attach one end of it to the I.V. tubing (as shown).

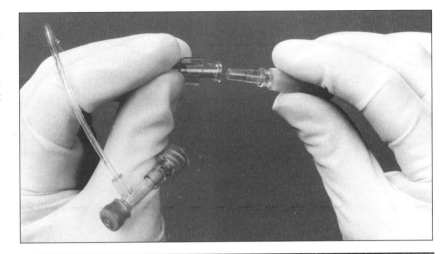

Open the slide clamp (as shown). Now you're ready to connect the luer-lock tip to the venipuncture device. Remove the tip's protective cap, and carefully connect the tip to the venipuncture device. Secure the connector with tape. As needed, I.V. medication can be administered through the latex injection port of the T-connector. Finally, document your actions on the patient's medication record.

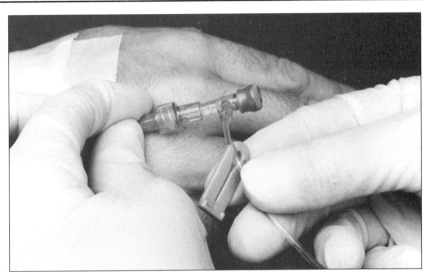

Monitoring the infusion

During the infusion, frequently check that the medication in the secondary I.V. line is infusing at the desired rate and over the desired time. When a continuous secondary infusion finishes, the primary infusion will continue. Likewise, when a piggyback solution finishes infusing, the primary infusion will resume. In either case, adjust the primary I.V. solution drip rate, as needed, when the secondary infusion finishes. If you're using an infusion pump, reset the rate or volume as needed.

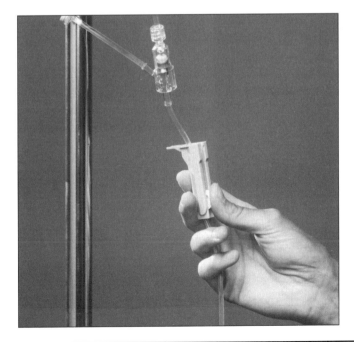

If you'll be reusing the tubing from the secondary infusion set on the same patient, close the clamp on the tubing. Then replace the used needle with a new one, or leave it securely taped or locked in the injection port. According to hospital policy, label the tubing with the time it was first used (as shown). Also, leave the empty secondary solution container in place until you replace it with a new one. Change this tubing according to hospital policy (usually every 48 to 72 hours). Inspect the injection port for leakage with each use. Change the port more often if needed.

If you won't be reusing the tubing from the secondary line, discard it appropriately along with the empty solution container.

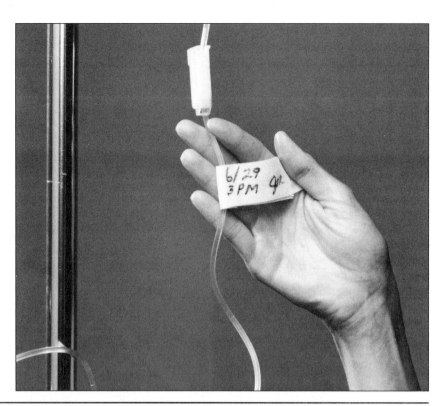

Finally, record the amounts and types of drug and I.V. solution on the intake and output and medication records. Note the date, time, duration, and rate of infusion, and the patient's responses, where applicable.

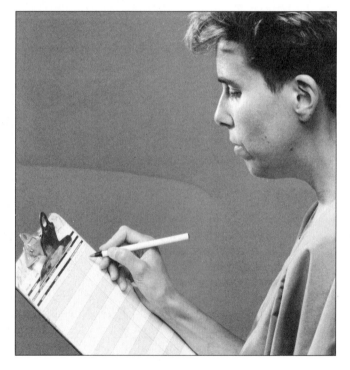

GIVING AN I.V. BOLUS INJECTION

Commonly called *I.V. push,* an I.V. bolus injection allows rapid drug delivery and a maximum, or *peak,* drug level in the patient's bloodstream immediately. Used in emergencies, the technique also allows administration of a drug that can't be diluted—for example, phenytoin, digoxin, furosemide, diazoxide, diazepam, many chemotherapeutic drugs, and diagnostic contrast media.

Usually, you'll give a bolus injection directly into an existing peripheral primary I.V. line, an existing intermittent infusion device, or a vein. You may also use the technique to give a drug through an existing central venous line or vascular access port. Because a drug given by I.V. bolus takes effect rapidly, you'll need to monitor your patient carefully for such adverse reactions as cardiac arrhythmias.

ENSURING PATIENT SAFETY

For certain drugs, the manufacturer supplies specific administration directions, such as the appropriate injection rate. If you don't have such directions, keep these precautions in mind:

• Don't give an I.V. bolus when you need to dilute a drug—an antibiotic or a vitamin, for example—in a large-volume parenteral solution before it enters the bloodstream.

• Avoid an I.V. bolus whenever the rapid administration of a drug, such as potassium chloride, could be life-threatening.

• Finish each bolus injection by recording the type and amount of drug given and the administration times on the patient's medication record. Record all I.V. solutions used to dilute the drug and flush the line on the patient's intake and output record.

• Keep in mind that drug tolerance declines in patients with decreased cardiac output, diminished urine output, pulmonary congestion, or systemic edema. To compensate, you'll need to dilute the prescribed drug more than usual and administer it at a slower rate.

To give a bolus injection through an existing peripheral I.V. line or an intermittent infusion device, you'll need the prescribed medication in a syringe with an attached 20G or 22G 1″ needle, alcohol sponges, two syringes (usually 3-ml) filled with 0.9% sodium chloride solution with attached 20G or 22G 1″ needles, gloves, and the patient's medication record. Depending on hospital policy, you may need another 3-ml syringe with an attached 20G or 22G 1″ needle filled with heparin flush solution.

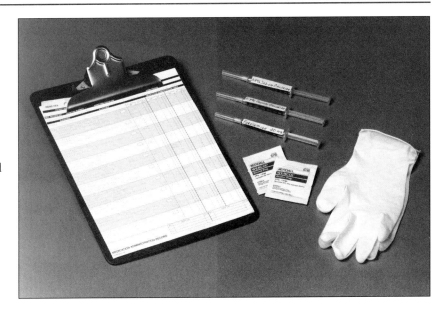

To administer a bolus injection directly into a vein, obtain a winged venipuncture device, a tourniquet, alcohol sponges or povidone-iodine sponges, two syringes filled with 0.9% sodium chloride solution, one syringe filled with the prescribed medication, 1″ hypoallergenic tape or an adhesive bandage, sterile 2″ × 2″ gauze pads, gloves, and the patient's medication record.

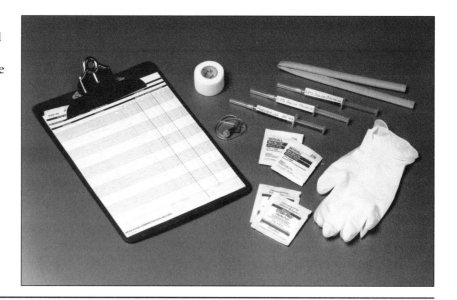

Compare the order on the patient's medication record with the doctor's order. Take the prepared medication, flush solutions, and other equipment to the patient's bedside, and explain the procedure to him. Verify the patient's identity by asking him his name and comparing the name, room number, and bed number on his identification bracelet with the same information on the medication record.

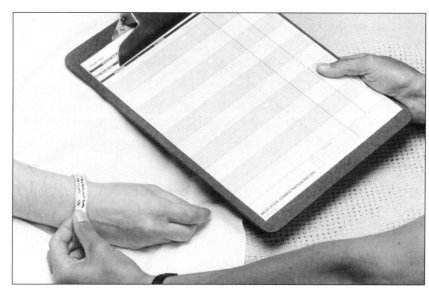

Delivering an I.V. bolus through a peripheral I.V. line

Check the compatibility of the medication with the I.V. solution. If they're compatible, put on gloves and close the flow clamp on the existing I.V. line. Clean the Y-port closest to the venipuncture site with an alcohol sponge or a povidone-iodine sponge. Insert the syringe's needle into the Y-port and inject the medication.

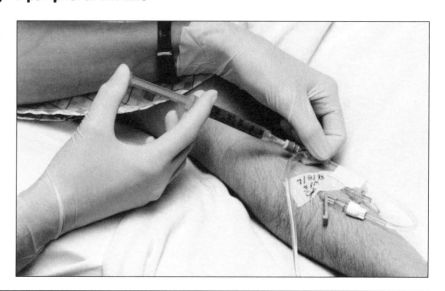

After injecting the medication, remove the needle from the Y-port, open the flow clamp on the I.V. line, and readjust the primary solution flow rate as prescribed. Document the procedure.

▶ *Clinical tip:* If you're delivering a drug that's incompatible with the primary I.V. solution, consult the pharmacist and check with the drug manufacturer for directions. You may be able to flush the line with 2 to 3 ml of 0.9% sodium chloride solution, administer the drug, again flush the line and then restart the flow of the primary I.V. solution. If you can't do this, insert a venipuncture device to deliver the medication, or use a T-connector.

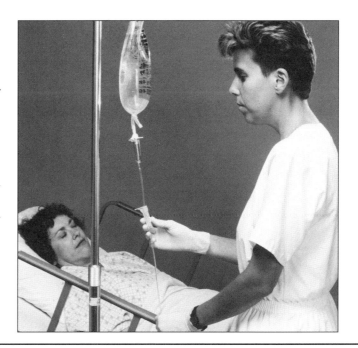

Delivering an I.V. bolus through an intermittent infusion device

Put on gloves. Clean the infusion port of the intermittent infusion device with an alcohol sponge. Verify the device's patency and proper placement in the vein by inserting the needle of one syringe filled with 0.9% sodium chloride solution and aspirating for blood. If no blood appears, apply a tourniquet above the site for about 1 minute. Aspirate again. If blood still doesn't appear, remove the tourniquet and inject the sodium chloride solution slowly. Stop if you feel resistance, indicating an occlusion. In this case, insert a new intermittent infusion device.

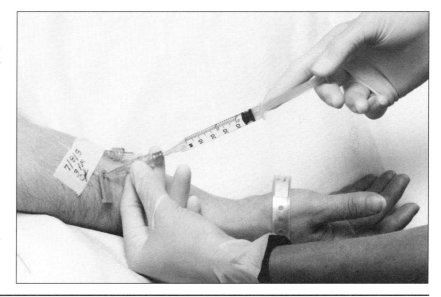

Once you aspirate blood, slowly inject the 0.9% sodium chloride solution and observe for signs of infiltration (puffiness or pain at the site). If infiltration occurs, remove and reinsert the intermittent infusion device. After flushing, withdraw the syringe and the needle.

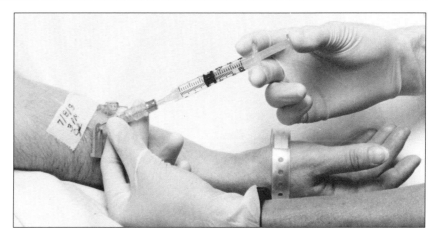

Insert the needle of the medication-filled syringe into the injection port of the intermittent infusion device. Inject the medication (as shown) at the appropriate rate; then remove this needle. Insert the needle of the other syringe filled with 0.9% sodium chloride solution into the injection port. Inject the solution to flush the drug through the intermittent infusion device, and remove this needle. Document the procedure on the patient's medication record. Record the amount of I.V. solution used to dilute the medication and to flush the line on the intake and output record.

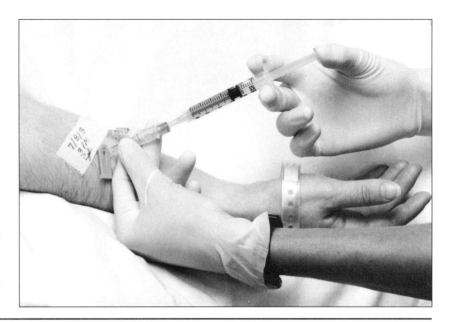

Delivering an I.V. bolus directly into a vein

Select the largest vein suitable for an injection. The larger the vein, the more the drug must be diluted to minimize vascular irritation. Apply a tourniquet above the injection site to distend the site.

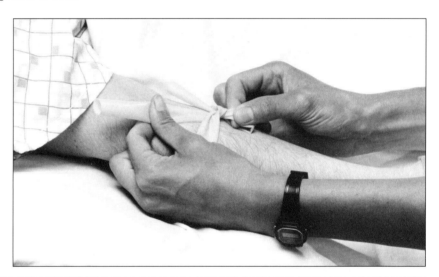

Put on gloves. Clean the injection site with an alcohol sponge or a povidone-iodine sponge. Work outward from the site in a circular motion to prevent recontaminating the site with skin bacteria.

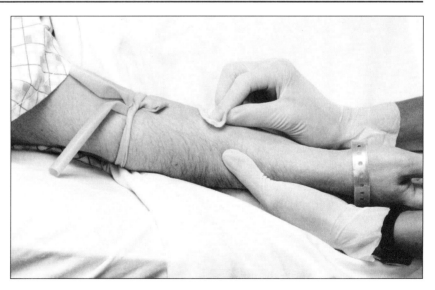

Using the winged venipuncture device, insert the needle, bevel side up, into the vein. Tape the wings in place with a single piece of tape. Depending on the size of the needle, you may or may not see blood in the tubing.

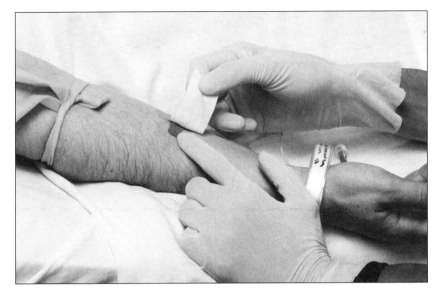

Attach a syringe filled with 0.9% sodium chloride solution to the venipuncture device. Pull back on the plunger to further check for blood backflow.

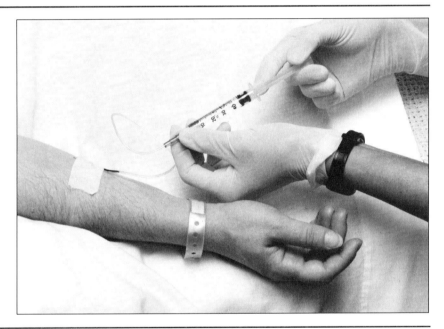

Once blood flows back into the tubing, remove the tourniquet and slowly inject the 0.9% sodium chloride solution into the vein, observing for signs of infiltration. Then remove this syringe from the tubing and attach the medication-filled syringe to the winged venipuncture device. Inject the medication at the appropriate rate (as shown).

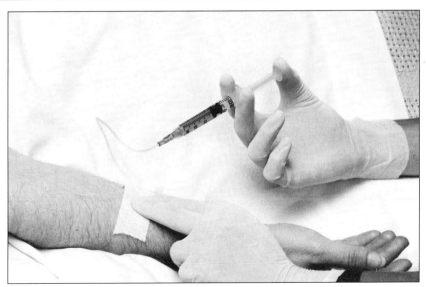

Remove the used medication syringe, and attach the second syringe filled with 0.9% sodium chloride solution. Flush the winged venipuncture device with this solution to ensure delivery of all the medication into the vein.

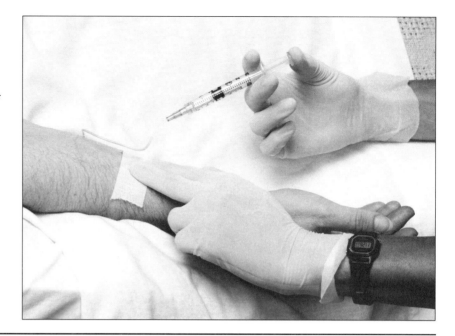

Alternatively, you can attach a 3-ml syringe filled with 0.9% sodium chloride solution to one side of a three-way stopcock and the medication-filled syringe to another side of the stopcock. Then attach the stopcock to the venipuncture device. You can check for blood backflow, inject the medication, and flush the venipuncture device by turning the stopcock to the appropriate positions.

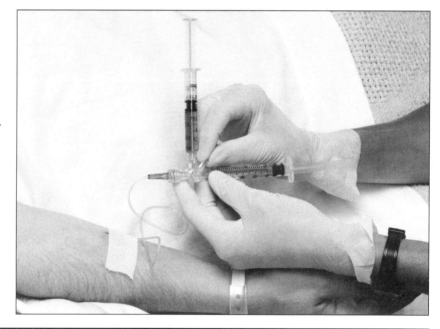

Remove the venipuncture device from the vein, and cover the site with a sterile 2″ × 2″ gauze pad. Apply pressure to the site for at least 3 minutes to prevent a hematoma from forming. After bleeding stops, secure the gauze with tape or an adhesive bandage. Finally, record the type and amount of drug given and the times of administration on the patient's medication record.

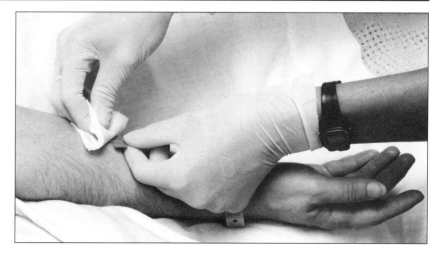

USING A CONTROLLED-RELEASE INFUSION SYSTEM

IVAC Corporation's controlled-release infusion system (CRIS) offers an alternative way to administer secondary drugs through a primary I.V. line. Connected to the I.V. line between the primary container and the administration set, this adapter-like device allows you to administer a drug dose without using a minibag and a piggyback administration set. You attach a single-dose vial to the CRIS adapter's spike and turn the valve handle toward the vial. The primary infusion flows into the vial and mixes with the drug; the mixture then flows down the line to the patient. The CRIS works with any I.V. solution container and any primary set. Use it with unvented I.V. tubing and liquid or reconstituted drugs in single-dose vials (from 5 to 20 ml).

Besides being easy to operate, the CRIS adapter can save you time. When using it, you needn't interrupt the primary flow to administer a secondary drug, and you don't have to flush the I.V. tubing between drug deliveries. Because you don't need additional solution containers, you can modify the patient's fluid intake easily and save the time you'd spend priming secondary sets, adjusting and readjusting flow rates, and handling secondary containers. What's more, the adapter saves the storage space you'd use for minibags and secondary I.V. sets.

To use the CRIS adapter, the patient must have a primary I.V. line in place. Gather the additional equipment you'll need, including the CRIS adapter itself, liquid or reconstituted medication in a single-dose vial (in quantities ranging from 5 to 20 ml, as ordered), alcohol sponges, and the patient's medication record. Depending on the situation, you may also need time tape, an infusion pump, or unvented tubing.

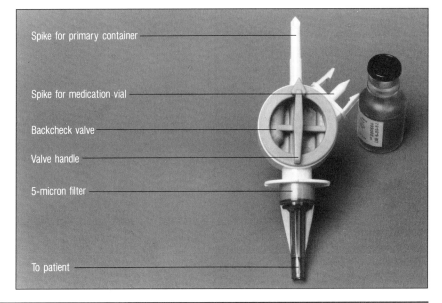

Spike for primary container

Spike for medication vial

Backcheck valve

Valve handle

5-micron filter

To patient

Compare the order on the medication record with the doctor's order on the patient's chart. Then go to the patient's room, ask him his name, and compare the name, room number, and bed number on the medication record with the information on the patient's identification bracelet. Explain the procedure to the patient. Check that his I.V. setup has unvented tubing (as shown). If the setup has vented tubing, replace it with the appropriate apparatus.

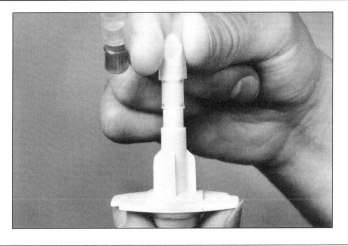

Contributors to this section include *Mary Jane McDevitt, RN, BS,* an oncology nurse at Mercy Catholic Medical Center, Fitzgerald Mercy Division, Darby, Pa., and *Denise Salvo, RN,C, MSN, CCRN,* an instructor at Widener University, Chester, Pa. The publisher thanks *Doylestown (Pa.) Hospital* and *IVAC Corp.,* San Diego, for their help.

To install the CRIS adapter on the patient's I.V. line, push—don't twist—the spike of the administration set into the adapter's lower port. Pick up the single-dose vial of medication (as ordered) and an alcohol sponge.

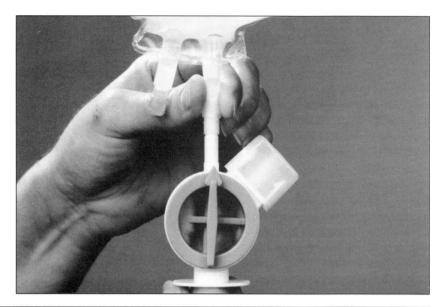

Remove the temporary cover and clean the vial's diaphragm with the alcohol sponge. With a twisting motion, remove the protective cover from the spike, and impale the vial on the spike.

▶ *Clinical tip:* If you encounter resistance, puncture the diaphragm with a needle to release air.

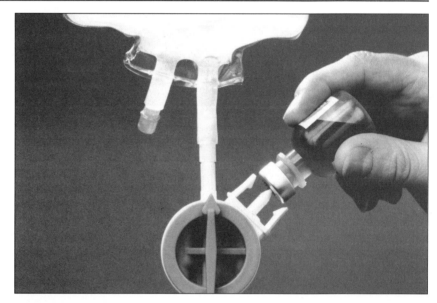

Make sure that the primary container of I.V. solution holds at least 60 ml of fluid (the volume needed to deliver the dose and flush the system). Then, to begin drug delivery, turn the CRIS's valve handle toward the vial until you feel resistance. Click the valve into place in the 2 o'clock position. Calculate the flow rate and mark the primary container to indicate the amount that should be infused. Mark a time tape or set the infusion pump appropriately.

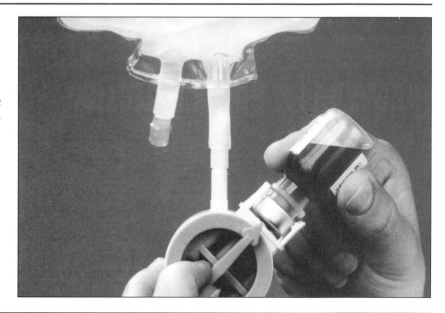

After the medication is delivered, leave the vial in place and keep the valve handle in the 2 o'clock position until the patient needs another dose. (Note that the primary infusion flows through the vial; therefore, the vial doesn't empty.) Leaving the vial in place keeps the vial's spike sterile.

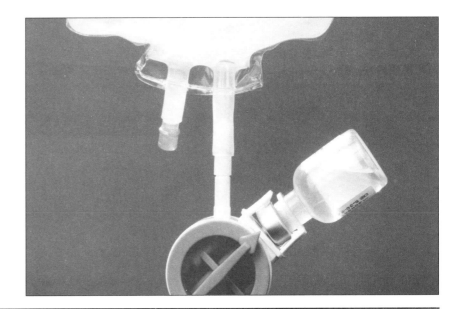

Before giving another drug dose, make sure that the primary I.V. container holds at least 60 ml of fluid. Then turn the valve handle to the 12 o'clock position (as shown). Adjust the fluid level of the drip chamber, if necessary.

If the vial inadvertently becomes pressurized during drug reconstitution, if the drug produces gas, or if you squeeze the drip chamber with the valve in the 2 o'clock position, the backcheck valve will prevent reflux of the drug solution into the primary container.

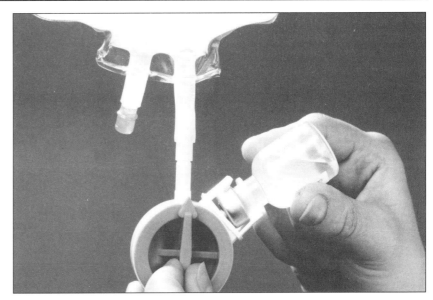

Remove the used medication vial and replace it with a new one (as shown). Turn the valve handle back to the 2 o'clock position. Adjust the flow rate, if necessary. Change the CRIS adapter when you change the administration set—every 48 hours or according to hospital policy.

▶ *Clinical tip:* You can use the CRIS adapter on a primary I.V. line while delivering another drug through a piggyback set.

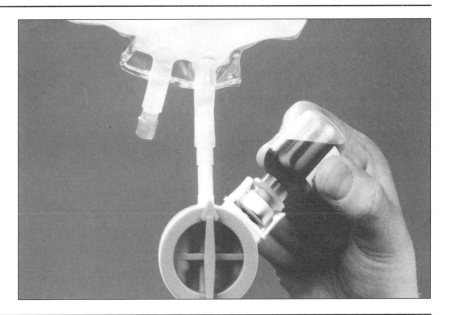

DELIVERING DRUGS WITH A SYRINGE PUMP

You may find a syringe pump useful when you're administering small volumes of medication intermittently or continuously. Able to deliver fluid very slowly, the syringe pump is ideal for pediatric and neonatal patients and for oncology departments, emergency departments, and labor and delivery settings.

Compact and portable, the syringe pump uses a disposable syringe with a 50-ml volume limit and operates on either alternating current (AC) or a rechargeable battery. Typically, a motor-driven lead screw or gear mechanism controls the syringe's plunger. The motor's speed determines how quickly the plunger moves and, in turn, the infusion rate. Keep in mind that the pump lacks an air detector, so make sure that you eliminate all air bubbles from the syringe, tubing, and needle before you start the infusion.

The following pages feature the IVAC 710 syringe pump. This unit is compatible with several types of 50-ml syringes and has an occlusion detection alarm.

Preparing the syringe pump

Assemble this equipment at the patient's bedside: the syringe pump, a sterile syringe extension set, a 50-ml syringe labeled and prefilled with the appropriate medication, a 20G 1″ needle, alcohol sponges, clean gloves, hypoallergenic tape, and the patient's medication record.

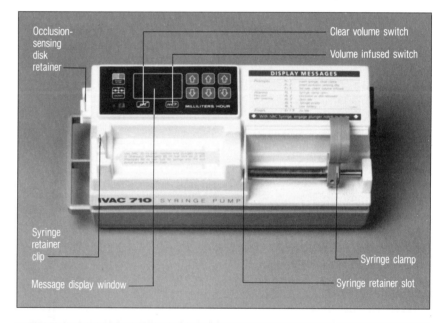

Occlusion-sensing disk retainer

Clear volume switch

Volume infused switch

Syringe retainer clip

Message display window

Syringe clamp

Syringe retainer slot

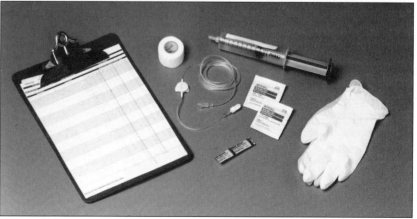

Pamela Kovach, RN, BSN, an independent nurse consultant for Springhouse Corporation, contributed to this section. The publisher thanks *Hill-Rom,* Batesville, Ind., and *IVAC Corp.,* San Diego, for their help.

Explain the procedure to the patient, and wash your hands. Confirm the patient's identity by asking him his name and comparing the name, room number, and bed number on his identification bracelet with the information on his medication record. Then match the label on the medication syringe with the drug ordered on the medication record.

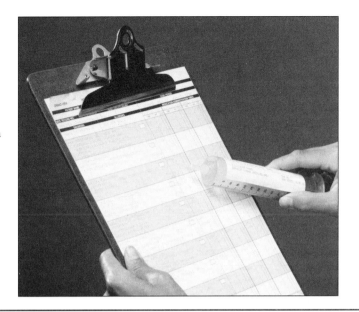

Connect the prefilled syringe to the extension set, using the set's female luer-lock. To prime the extension set, grasp the occlusion-sensing disk between your thumb and forefinger. Hold the membrane of the disk flat and rub your thumb over the membrane. With your other hand, push in the syringe's plunger. Tap the disk and push the plunger in again to completely expel trapped air.

▶ *Clinical tip:* Push the plunger to at least the 50-ml mark so that the syringe will fit into the clamp.

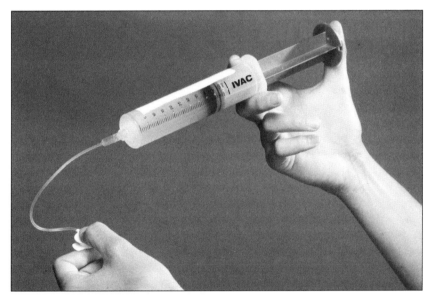

Turn on the pump by pressing the ON/OFF control. The pump will beep to confirm that it's functioning. When "Pr 1" appears in the message display window, open the syringe clamp and put the syringe (tip first) in the pump's cradle. Align the notch on the plunger with the track on the pump's case, and close the clamp over the end of the plunger (as shown). The next message to appear will read "Pr 2." This indicates that you may insert the occlusion-sensing disk into the disk retainer.

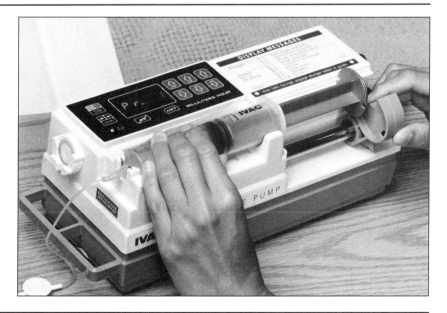

Insert the occlusion-sensing disk into the disk retainer on the end of the pump's case. Set the flow rate and the volume to be infused after the message "Pr 3" appears in the display window.

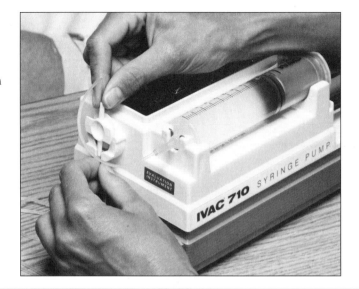

Press START/STOP or any of the MIL-LILITERS/HOUR controls to display the last rate selected. Press the appropriate MILLILITERS/HOUR controls (on this model they're up or down arrows) to enter the new flow rate (as shown). Press ML? (volume infused) to display the previous volume infused. Press ML? and ML (clear volume) to reset the volume infused to zero.

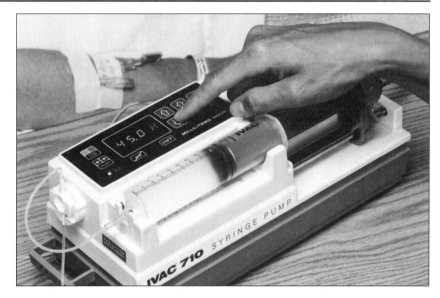

Infusing the drug

Put the pump on the same side of the bed as the I.V. setup to avoid crisscrossing I.V. lines over the patient. Put on gloves and attach a 20G needle to the male luer-lock of the I.V. extension set. Wipe the injection port with an alcohol sponge. Then insert the needle into the patient's I.V. port or intermittent infusion device (as shown). Secure the needle and tubing using hypoallergenic tape, according to hospital policy. Then press START/STOP to begin the infusion. Periodically check the patient's I.V. line for patency and the site for infiltration.

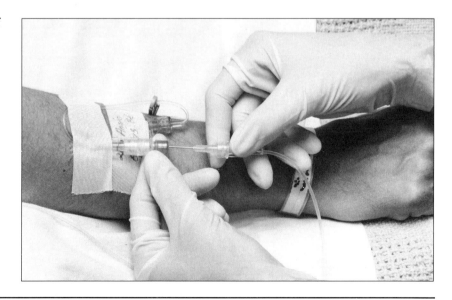

To change the rate or temporarily stop the infusion, press START/ STOP. A flashing "H" will appear on the right side of the message display window, and the pump will sound a repeated click, indicating that it has stopped infusing. The pump will stay on hold for 2 minutes. To change the rate, press the MILLILITERS/HOUR arrows. Then restart the infusion by pressing START/STOP.

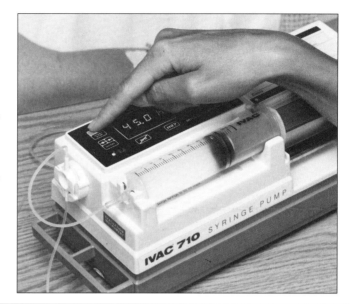

When the syringe is almost empty, the infusion indicator (located on the right side of the message display window) will change to half-size and a repeated double click tone will sound. To continue the infusion, put the pump on hold and replace the syringe. When all of the ordered medication has been infused, turn off the pump and disconnect the tubing from the patient. If the patient has an intermittent infusion device, flush it according to hospital policy. Document the procedure.

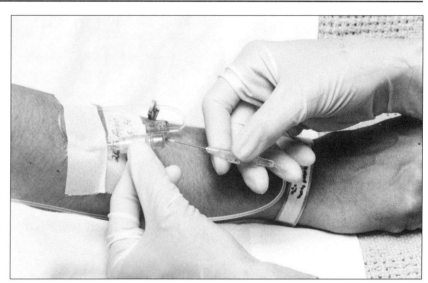

 TROUBLESHOOTING

Correcting syringe pump problems

PROBLEM	POSSIBLE CAUSE	SOLUTION
Battery light flashing and audible alarm	Battery losing its charge	Plug the pump into a wall outlet, and turn the power off and on. You may have to wait several minutes before the pump will function.
Battery light flashing while operating on AC	Blown fuse or pump malfunction	Check the fuses. If you replace the fuse and it blows again, call for service.
No display and audible alarm when turning pump on	Pump battery too low	Plug the pump into a wall outlet. You may have to wait several minutes before the pump will function.
No display and audible alarm with pump on hold	The 2-minute hold limit passed without an intervention, such as opening the clamp or changing one of the controls.	Press START/STOP once to silence the alarm and again when you're ready to restart the infusion.

GIVING DRUGS THROUGH AN IMPLANTED V.A.P.

Surgically placed beneath a patient's skin, an implanted vascular access port (VAP) permits intermittent long-term delivery of medications (including chemotherapeutic agents), I.V. fluids, total parenteral nutrition, or blood products through a central venous line. You can also use the device to obtain blood samples.

A VAP is used most commonly when an external central venous (CV) catheter isn't desirable for long-term I.V. therapy. (See *Understanding VAPs.*) It also offers several advantages, including minimal activity restrictions and few self-care measures for the patient to learn and perform. The site doesn't require a dressing (perhaps only a small adhesive bandage after an infusion) except when used for continuous

or prolonged infusions. The risk of infection is also lower because the device has no exposed exit site. One- and two-piece units with single or double lumens are available.

However, a VAP also has some disadvantages. Because the device is implanted, the patient may find it difficult to manage, particularly if she will use it at home to administer medication or fluids daily or frequently. And because using the device requires inserting a needle through subcutaneous tissue, the patient may require a local anesthetic.

Implanted VAPs are contraindicated in patients who can't tolerate other implanted devices and in those who may develop an allergic reaction.

Understanding VAPs

An implanted vascular access port (VAP) functions much like a long-term central venous line, except that it has no external parts. The attached indwelling catheter is tunneled through the subcutaneous tissue until its tip enters a central vein (the subclavian vein, for example).

The port itself consists of a small reservoir, which may be made of titanium, stainless steel, or molded plastic. A self-sealing silicone rubber septum designed to withstand multiple punctures provides entry to the reservoir and seals it.

Completely covered by the patient's skin, the VAP reduces the risk of extrinsic contamination and may be preferred because it provides greater freedom and doesn't alter the patient's body image. What's more, it requires less routine catheter care than other central lines.

VAPs come in two basic designs: top-entry and side-entry. In a top-entry device, the needle enters the port perpendicular to the reservoir. In a side-entry device, the needle enters the port through the septum, which lies nearly parallel to the reservoir. (A needle stop prevents the needle from coming out the other side.)

Top-entry VAP

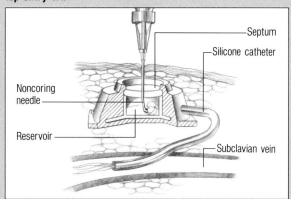

Side-entry VAP

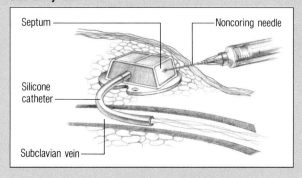

Contributors to this section include *Mary Jane McDevitt, RN, BS,* an oncology nurse at Mercy Catholic Medical Center, Fitzgerald Mercy Division, Darby, Pa., and *Denise Salvo, RN,C, MSN, CCRN,* an instructor at Widener University, Chester, Pa. The publisher thanks *Hill-Rom,* Batesville, Ind., and *Reganes, Inc.,* Tarpon Springs, Fla., for their help.

Using a VAP

Gather this equipment: a noncoring needle of appropriate type and gauge (usually a straight or right-angle Huber needle), extension tubing with clamp (this equipment may already be attached to the Huber needle), gloves, two masks, alcohol swabs, povidone-iodine swabs, two 10-ml syringes prefilled with 0.9% sodium chloride solution, a 5 ml syringe prefilled with heparin flush solution, a local anesthetic (such as 1% or 2% lidocaine), a tuberculin syringe, sterile drapes, sterile 2″ × 2″ gauze pads, and the patient's medication record. If you'll be using the VAP within 72 hours of insertion, you'll also need an ice pack.

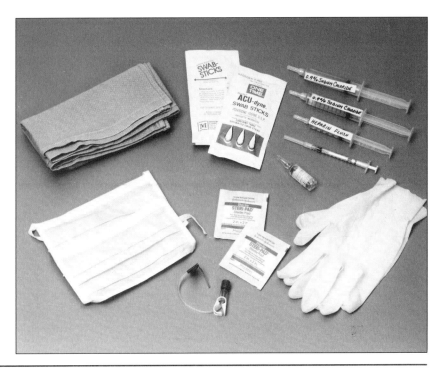

Take the equipment to the patient's bedside. Identify the patient by asking her name and checking her identification bracelet. Explain the procedure and wash your hands. Put on a mask and have the patient wear one too. Also put on gloves. Inspect the area around the port for signs of infection and skin breakdown.

▶ *Clinical tip:* The VAP can be used immediately after placement, although some edema and tenderness may persist for about 72 hours. This makes the device initially difficult to palpate and slightly uncomfortable for the patient. Place an ice pack over the area for several minutes to alleviate discomfort from the needle puncture.

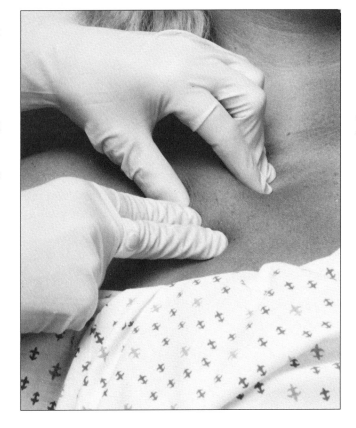

Clean the area with an alcohol swab. Start at the center of the port and work outward for 4″ to 5″ (10 to 13 cm), using a firm, circular motion (as shown). Repeat this procedure two more times, using a new alcohol swab each time. Then clean the area the same way with the povidone-iodine swabs. Remove any excess povidone-iodine by dabbing the area with a sterile gauze pad. If your hospital policy calls for a local anesthetic, check the patient's record for possible allergies. As indicated, numb the insertion site by injecting 0.1 ml of lidocaine (without epinephrine) using a tuberculin syringe.

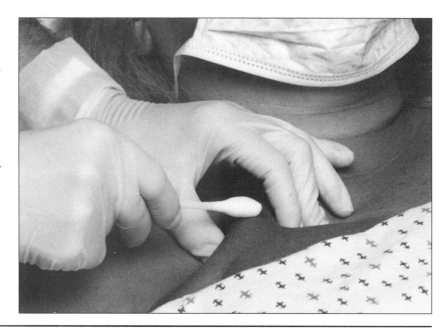

Place a sterile drape around the patient. Attach one of the 10-ml prefilled syringes containing 0.9% sodium chloride solution to the end of the extension tubing attached to the noncoring needle. Fill the tubing with the solution and close the clamp.

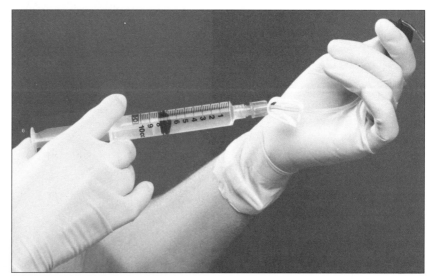

Using a top-entry VAP

To use a top-entry port, palpate the area over the port to locate the port septum. Anchor the port between the thumb and first two fingers of your nondominant hand. Use your dominant hand to aim the noncoring needle at the center of the VAP and insert it perpendicular to the port's septum. Push the needle through the skin and septum until you reach the bottom of the reservoir.

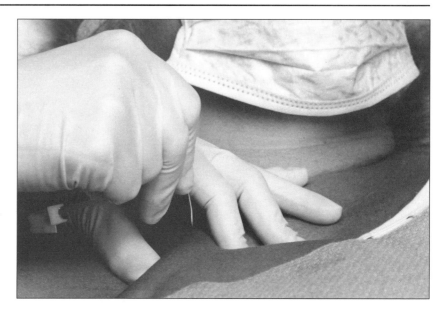

Check for correct needle placement by aspirating for blood return. If you obtain blood, inject 5 ml of heparin flush solution. If you can't obtain blood, remove the needle and aspirate again.

▶ *Clinical tip:* Inability to obtain blood suggests that the catheter leading from the port is lodged against the vessel wall. Ask the patient to raise her arms, perform Valsalva's maneuver, or change position to free the catheter. If this doesn't work, notify the doctor; a fibrin sleeve on the distal end of the catheter may be occluding the opening.

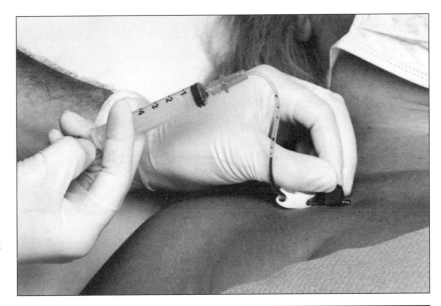

Flush the VAP with the other syringe containing 0.9% sodium chloride solution. Then clamp the extension tubing. If you detect swelling, or if the patient reports pain at the site, remove the needle and notify the doctor.

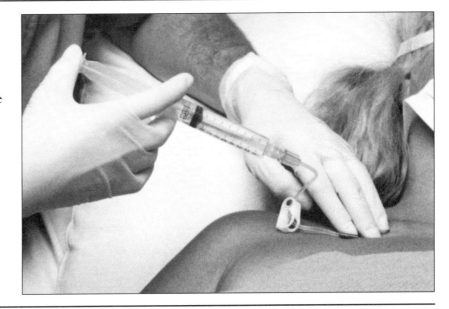

Using a side-entry VAP

To use a side-entry port, follow the same procedure as with a top-entry port. However, insert the needle parallel to the reservoir instead of perpendicular to it.

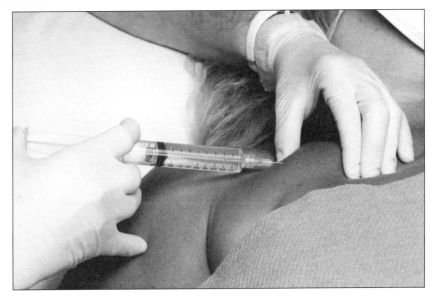

Administering a bolus injection through a VAP

In addition to the equipment required to use the VAP, you'll need a syringe containing the prescribed medication, two 10-ml syringes prefilled with 0.9% sodium chloride solution, a 5-ml syringe prefilled with heparin flush solution, and the patient's medication record.

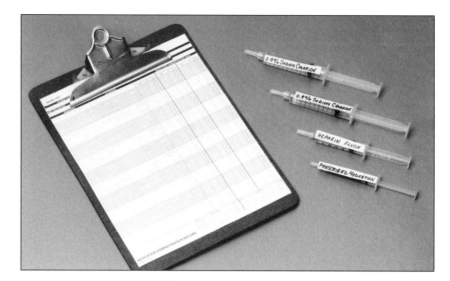

Verify the medication order on the medication record and the patient's chart. If you haven't already done so, attach a syringe filled with 0.9% sodium chloride to the extension set. Flush the set and the VAP. Then connect the medication syringe to the extension set.

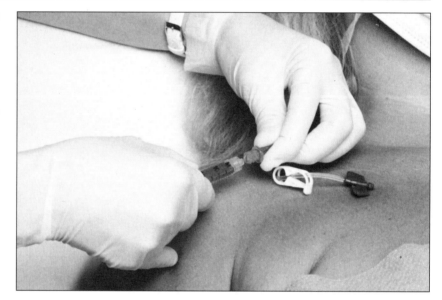

Open the clamp and inject the drug as ordered. Examine the skin surrounding the needle for signs of infiltration, such as swelling or tenderness. If you note these signs, stop the injection and notify the doctor.

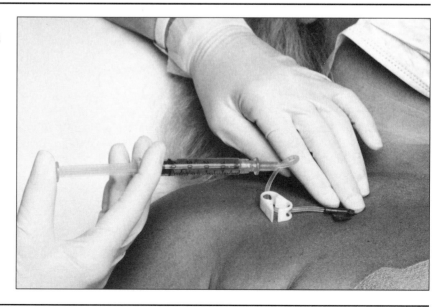

After completing the injection, clamp the extension set and remove the medication syringe. Attach the other syringe with 0.9% sodium chloride solution, and flush the set and the VAP with 5 ml of the solution. Perform this step after each drug injection to minimize possible drug incompatibility reactions. Also, flush with heparin flush solution, if your hospital's policy requires it. After flushing, remove the needle and document the procedure.

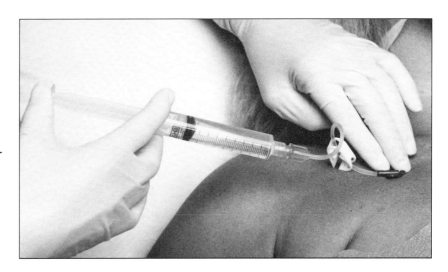

Administering a continuous infusion through a VAP

In addition to the equipment required to use the VAP, you'll need the prescribed I.V. solution or medication, an I.V. administration set, a 10-ml syringe filled with 0.9% sodium chloride solution, povidone-iodine ointment, and the patient's medication record. You'll also need a transparent semipermeable dressing and possibly a filter.

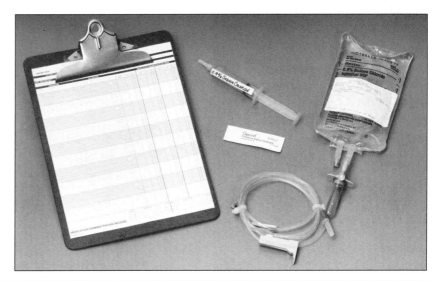

Verify the medication against the patient's medication record. Connect the administration set, and secure the connections with sterile tape, if necessary. Unclamp the extension set, open the clamp on the administration set (as shown), and begin the infusion.

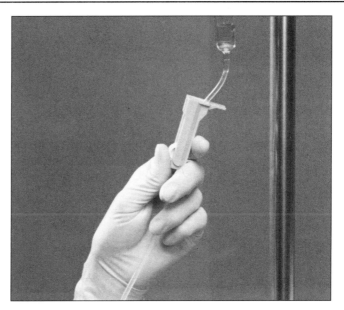

Depending on your hospital's policy, you may apply a small amount
of povidone-iodine ointment to the
insertion site (as shown); then apply a transparent semipermeable
dressing over the entire site.

▶ *Clinical tip:* If the needle
hub isn't flush with the
skin, place a folded, sterile
2″ × 2″ gauze pad under the hub.
Then apply Steri-Strips across it.
Secure the needle and tubing with
a chevron-taping technique.

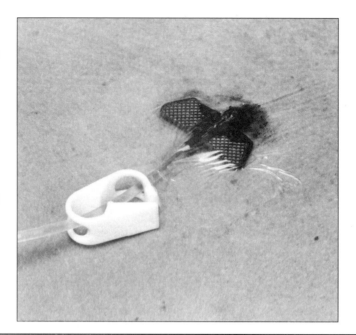

Examine the site carefully for infiltration. If you note infiltration
or if the patient complains of
stinging, burning, or pain at the
site, clamp the extension tubing,
discontinue the infusion, and notify the doctor. Dispose of all
soiled supplies and used equipment appropriately. Wash your
hands and document the procedure.

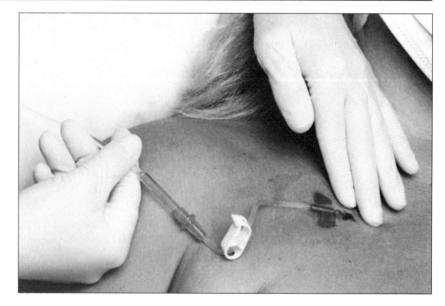

GIVING DRUGS THROUGH AN ENDOTRACHEAL TUBE

When an I.V. line isn't readily available in a life-threatening emergency, you can administer drugs safely and effectively through an endotracheal (ET) tube. You'll use this route only until an I.V. line can be established.

Endotracheally delivered drugs take effect more rapidly than those given by I.M. injection (another possible emergency route) because the pulmonary alveoli provide a large surface area for drug absorption. Pulmonary circulation propels blood to the left side of the heart, ensuring rapid, central drug dissemination. However, only a few drugs, such as atropine, epinephrine, and lidocaine, can adequately penetrate the pulmonary surface.

The duration of action is usually longer with ET tube delivery than with I.V. administration because the alveoli sustain absorption—known as the "depot effect." Therefore, you'll need to adjust subsequent doses and monitor I.V. infusions to guard against adverse effects.

Take the needed equipment to the patient's bedside: gloves, a stethoscope, a hand-held resuscitation bag, the prescribed drug, a syringe with a needle, and sterile distilled water or sterile 0.9% sodium chloride solution, as ordered.

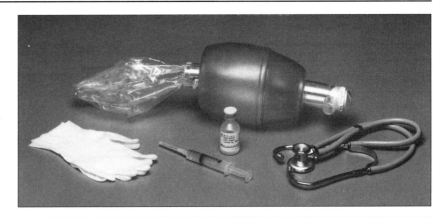

If possible, explain the procedure to the patient. Then wash your hands. If you haven't already done so, calculate the drug dose. Then dilute the drug with 5 to 10 ml of sterile distilled water or sterile 0.9% sodium chloride solution, as directed.

Note that the absorption of a drug diluted by water exceeds that of a drug diluted by 0.9% sodium chloride solution. However, a drug diluted by water tends to lower the partial pressure of arterial oxygen.

▶ *Clinical tip:* According to the American Heart Association's guidelines for Advanced Cardiac Life Support, the drug dose given through an ET tube should be 2 to 2½ times the recommended I.V. dose.

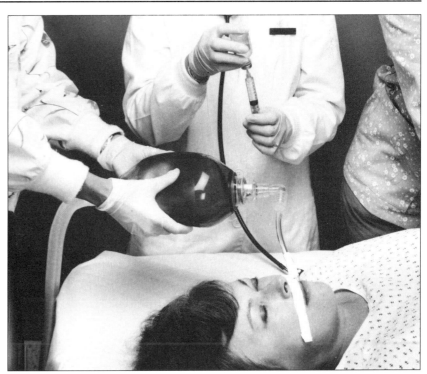

Mary Jane McDevitt, RN, BS, and *Karen Landis, RN, MS, CCRN,* contributed to this section. Ms. McDevitt is an oncology nurse at Mercy Catholic Medical Center, Fitzgerald Mercy Division, Darby, Pa. Ms. Landis is a pulmonary clinical nurse specialist at Lehigh Valley Hospital, Allentown, Pa. The publisher thanks *Doylestown (Pa.) Hospital* and *Hill-Rom,* Batesville, Ind., for their help.

Move the patient into a supine position with her head level with or slightly higher than her trunk. Put on clean gloves. Then auscultate the patient's lungs with a stethoscope while you ventilate her, to check the ET tube's position.

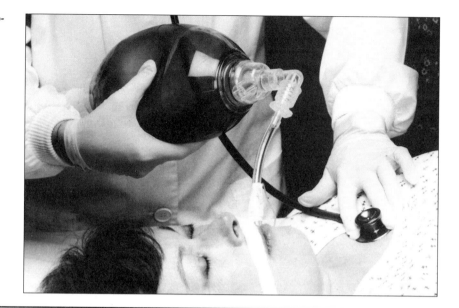

After confirming that the ET tube is properly positioned, provide three to five ventilations with the hand-held resuscitation bag. Then remove the bag from the ET tube (as shown).

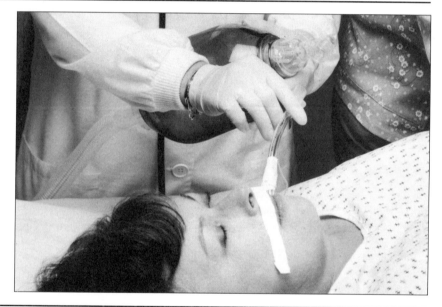

Next, remove the needle from the syringe, and insert the tip of the syringe into the ET tube. Rapidly instill the drug deep into the tube.

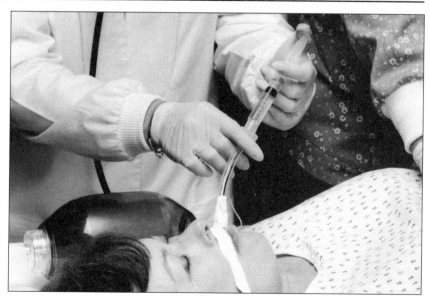

Place your thumb briefly over the ET tube after instilling the drug. This helps to minimize drug reflux.

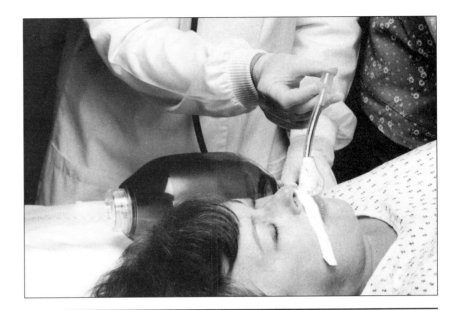

Reattach the resuscitation bag to the ET tube and provide five or six brisk ventilations (as shown). Doing so will propel the drug into the lungs, provide the patient with additional oxygen, and clear the ET tube. Monitor the patient's response to the medication. Be sure to dispose of the syringe correctly and document the procedure.

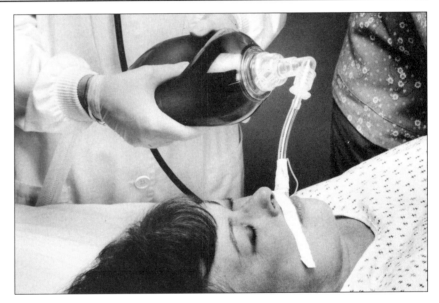

Reviewing endotracheal drugs and doses

Use this chart to help determine endotracheal drug doses in an emergency. Keep in mind that endotracheal doses are calculated by multiplying the usual I.V. dose 2 to 2½ times and that the drug should be diluted in 10 ml of sterile 0.9% sodium chloride solution or sterile distilled water, as prescribed. The endotracheal dose is provided below with the usual I.V. dose indicated in parentheses for reference.

DRUG	INDICATION	ENDOTRACHEAL DOSE	SPECIAL CONSIDERATIONS
Atropine	Symptomatic bradycardia or asystole	1 to 2.5 mg diluted in 10 ml of sterile 0.9% sodium chloride solution or sterile distilled water (0.5 to 1 mg I.V.)	• Monitor the patient's electrocardiogram continuously. • Atropine may cause tachycardia. Use cautiously in patients with cardiac ischemia or myocardial infarction because tachycardia increases myocardial oxygen consumption. • Full vagolytic doses (0.04 mg/kg) should be reserved for patients with asystole because of the risk of tachycardia.
Epinephrine (Adrenalin)	Cardiac arrest	2 to 2.5 mg diluted in 10 ml of sterile 0.9% sodium chloride solution or sterile distilled water (1 mg I.V.)	• Epinephrine has good bioavailability following endotracheal administration, but the optimal dose is unknown. • Researchers have compared high-dose epinephrine (5 mg I.V.) with the standard dose and have found no evidence of greater efficacy. As ordered, administer high-dose regimens only after standard doses have failed.
Lidocaine (Xylocaine 4%)	Ventricular tachycardia or ventricular fibrillation	2 to 3.75 mg/kg diluted in 10 ml of sterile 0.9% sodium chloride solution or sterile distilled water (1 to 1.5 mg/kg I.V.)	• Lidocaine is usually given by I.V. bolus followed by continuous I.V. infusion; only bolus therapy should be used in cardiac arrest. • Watch for signs of toxicity, such as metallic taste, somnolence, confusion, and seizures.

ASSISTING WITH AN INTRAPLEURAL INJECTION

Drugs may be injected through the chest wall via a catheter that has been inserted in the pleural space or through a chest tube that has been placed intrapleurally for drainage. Intrapleural administration (which scleroses the pleurae) provides superior chemotherapeutic effects, reduces drug toxicity, and maintains higher and longer-lasting pleural drug concentrations.

Increasingly, intrapleural administration is used to promote analgesia, treat spontaneous pneumothorax, resolve pleural effusions, and deliver chemotherapeutic drugs. Usually, drug delivery by chest tube is indicated for patients with empyema, pleural effusion, or pneumothorax; delivery by intrapleural catheter is indicated for all other patients. Drugs that are commonly administered by intrapleural injection include bleomycin, bupivacaine, doxycycline, and talc.

RISKS AND CONTRAINDICATIONS

Intrapleural injection can cause complications, such as pneumothorax or tension pneumothorax, if air accidentally enters the pleural cavity. Additional serious complications include chemical irritation of the pleurae and subsequent neutropenia or thrombocytopenia (or both) as well as pain and infection at the insertion site. However, meticulous skin preparation, strict aseptic technique, and sterile dressings usually prevent infection.

Drugs won't be given intrapleurally to a patient with fibrosis or adhesions (which impede drug infusion to the intended site), pleural inflammation, sepsis, or infection at the puncture site. Nor is intrapleural administration suitable for a patient with bullous emphysema or one who needs respiratory therapy with positive end-expiratory pressure, because the treatment may exacerbate an already compromised pulmonary condition.

To assist with intrapleural injection, take the following equipment to the patient's bedside: the prescribed medication in a 60-ml syringe, the patient's medication record, a rubber-tipped clamp (for clamping the chest tube), a face shield, a gown, gloves, and a sterile drape.

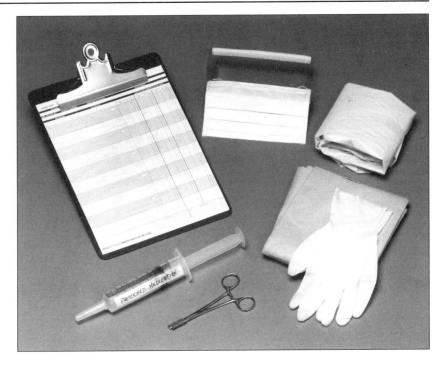

Explain the procedure to the patient. If required by hospital policy, make sure that he has signed a consent form. If the doctor prescribes a narcotic analgesic, put on gloves and administer it 30 minutes before the procedure.

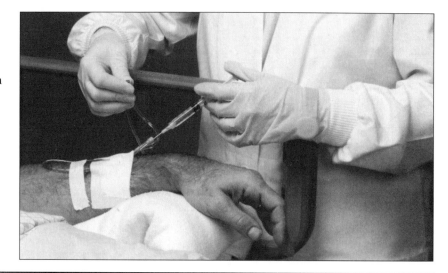

Verify the drug by comparing it to the patient's medication record. If the drug isn't already prepared, calculate the drug dose and dilute it with the correct amount of 0.9% sodium chloride solution or another diluent. Draw up the drug in a 60-ml syringe.

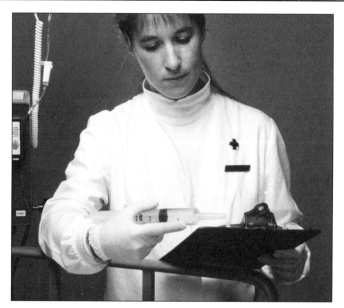

Position the patient on his side, with the affected side up. Clamp the chest tube.

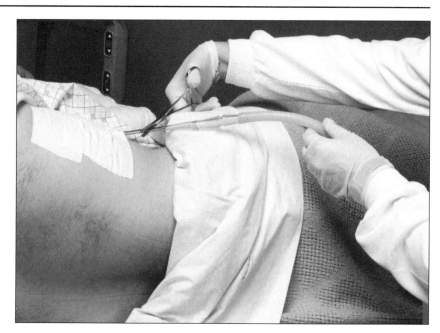

Put on a gown and face shield. The doctor will then aseptically place a sterile drape under the chest tube connection and disconnect the chest tube from the drainage system.

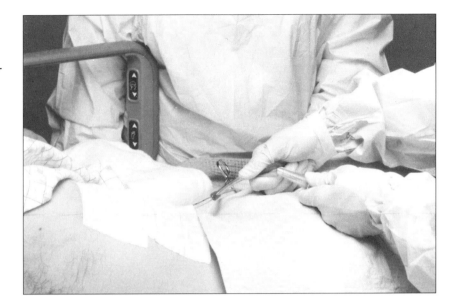

Next, the doctor will attach the medication-filled syringe to the chest tube, remove the clamp, and administer the medication (as shown).

After drug administration, you'll clamp the chest tube with the rubber-tipped clamp. Then close the clamp on the drainage tubing. Next, reconnect the chest tube to the drainage system (for added security).

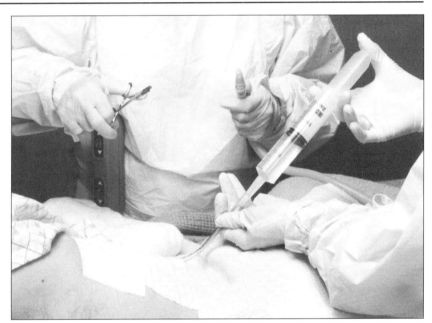

Ensure that the patient is as comfortable as possible. Have him remain on his unaffected side for 10 to 30 minutes, as tolerated, to help ensure that the medication circulates between the pleurae.

▶ *Clinical tip:* The longer this position is maintained, the better. However, the intense pain experienced by most patients usually prevents lengthy positioning.

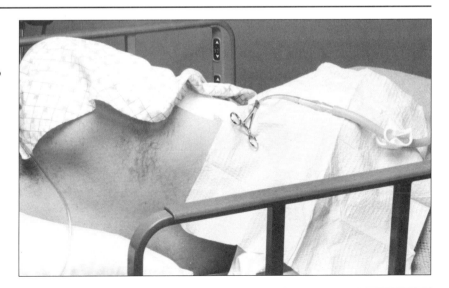

When the time has elapsed, help the patient into a supine position. Have him stay in this position for 10 to 30 minutes, as tolerated.

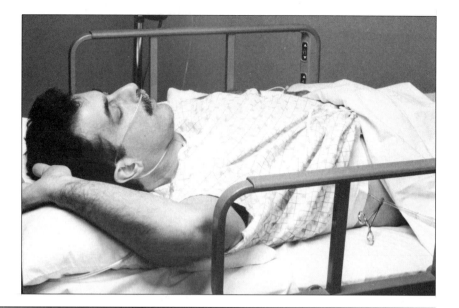

Next, help the patient into a prone position. Have him stay in this position for 10 to 30 minutes, as tolerated.

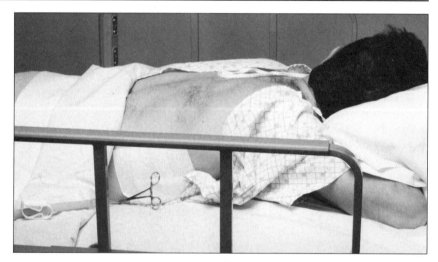

Help the patient into a sitting position. Have him stay in this position for 10 to 30 minutes, as tolerated. If he can't tolerate sitting, adjust the head of the bed (as shown) to an elevated position that he can endure for 10 to 30 minutes.

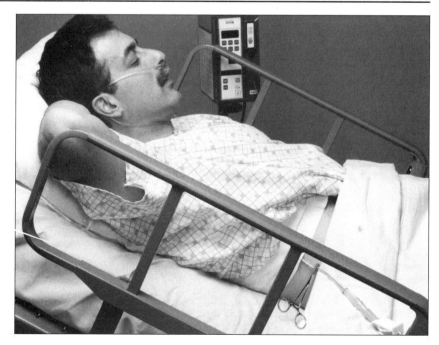

Now help the patient into Trende-
lenburg's position. Have him stay
in this position for 10 to 30 minutes, as tolerated.

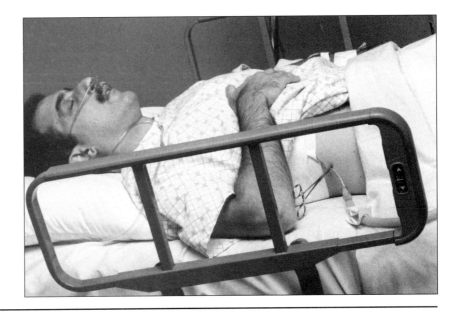

Position the patient on the affected
side for another 10 to 30 minutes.
If he reports pain during position
changes, the doctor may order another dose of narcotic analgesic.

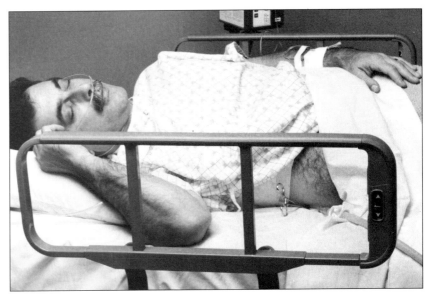

Finally, help the patient into a
comfortable position, usually semi-
Fowler's position. Remove the
clamp from the chest tube (as
shown).

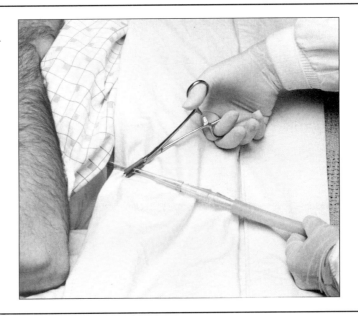

Unclamp the drainage tube and allow it to drain for 12 to 24 hours.
If ordered, connect the drainage
container to continuous wall suc-
tion. Document the procedure, including the medication provided
and the patient's tolerance of it.

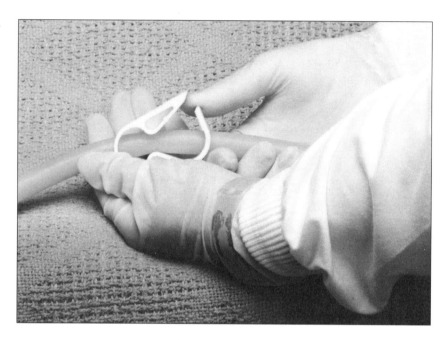

Reviewing intrapleural drugs and doses

DRUG	INDICATIONS	INTRAPLEURAL DOSE	SPECIAL CONSIDERATIONS
Bleomycin (Blenoxane)	Pleural effusions and lung cancer	One-time dose of 60 to 150 units; lifetime dosage shouldn't exceed 400 units (to prevent pulmonary toxicity)	• Assess respiratory function carefully before each treatment, especially in patients at high risk for pulmonary toxicity, such as those with dyspnea, bibasilar crackles, and a nonproductive cough. • Monitor the patient closely for 1 hour after treatment. • Monitor blood urea nitrogen level, creatinine clearance, and pulmonary function. • Arrange for chest X-rays before and during drug treatment. • Monitor the patient with lymphoma for possible allergic reactions.
Bupivacaine (Marcaine)	Postoperative pain from cholecystectomy, renal surgery, breast surgery, rib fractures, chest metastasis, or pancreatic cancer	Dosage shouldn't exceed 175 mg when administered alone or 225 mg when administered with epinephrine. Usually, dose shouldn't be repeated more than once every 3 hours. Daily dosage shouldn't exceed 400 mg.	• Observe the patient for adverse central nervous system effects, including dizziness, disorientation, blurred vision, drowsiness, and seizures. • Administer the drug cautiously to patients with hepatic dysfunction.
Doxycycline (Vibramycin)	Prevention of recurrent spontaneous pneumothorax and pleural effusion	One-time dose of 500 mg	• Inform the patient that this drug produces great discomfort, so he may receive a local anesthetic along with it as prescribed. • Tell the patient that the doctor will give him the injection.
Talc	Prevention of recurrent spontaneous pneumothorax and pleural effusion	One-time dose of 4 to 10 g	• Explain that the doctor will administer this drug after the patient undergoes general anesthesia. • Monitor the patient carefully for such adverse effects as fever, severe pain, hypertension, and tachycardia.

INDEX